Handbook of microscopic anatomy for the health sciences

Handbook of
microscopic anatomy
for the health sciences

ANNABELLE COHEN

Department of Biological Sciences
Staten Island Community College

with 99 illustrations

Original photomicrographs by

MARTIN H. ROSEN

Department of Biological Sciences
Staten Island Community College

THE C. V. MOSBY COMPANY

Saint Louis   1975

Copyright © 1975 by The C. V. Mosby Company

All rights reserved. No part of this book may be reproduced in any manner without written permission of the publisher.

Printed in the United States of America

Distributed in Great Britain by Henry Kimpton, London

Library of Congress Cataloging in Publication Data

Cohen, Annabelle, 1920-
  Handbook of microscopic anatomy for the health sciences.

  1. Histology. 2. Histology, Pathological.
II. Title. [DNLM: 1. Histology. 2. Neoplasms–
Pathology. QS504 C678h]
QM551.C62   616.9′92′07582   74-13572
ISBN 0-8016-1012-5

E/VH/VH 9 8 7 6 5 4 3 2 1

Preface

The science of histology (the study of tissues), particularly human histology, embraces a vast amount of data and uses a complex nomenclature derived from Greek and Latin roots. Most paraprofessional students have neither the time nor the inclination to study this valuable science in depth. Yet, in the course of their careers, they are frequently confronted by a broad spectrum of diseases caused by malignant transformations of normal cells and tissues. The abnormal cannot be understood without some comprehension of the normal. To function on an intelligent and effective level in a hospital atmosphere, nursing, technical and paramedical personnel should be familiar with the general features of microscopic anatomy, that is, with the structural organization of cells into tissues, tissues into organs, and organs into systems.

The purpose of this handbook is to bring this type of information in an organized and comprehensible form to students in the health sciences. The book is designed to emphasize only the most important aspects of the microscopic architecture of the human body but, at the same time, it is not intended to be merely a superficial treatment of the subject. The complex aspects are presented in as lucid and concise a manner as possible. The terminology, which is an integral part of the science, is carefully defined.

Although the study of abnormal tissues or tumors (histopathology) is usually outside the scope of a text of this nature, discussions and photomicrographs of commonly occurring malignant and benign tumors have been incorporated into the subject matter wherever practicable. It is hoped that this combined approach to normal and abnormal histology will give paraprofessionals the basic knowledge so vital to successful achievement in their chosen field.

Dr. Fidelio Jiminez, Chief of Pathology at the Veterans Hospital of Brooklyn, most generously contributed the microscopic sections of human tumors. I wish to express my sincere gratitude to Dr. Jiminez, to Dr. Philip Schain of the Department of Biological Sciences, Staten Island Community College, for his helpful advice, and to Mrs. Helen Bey for the use of her collection of Papanicolaou smears.

Annabelle Cohen

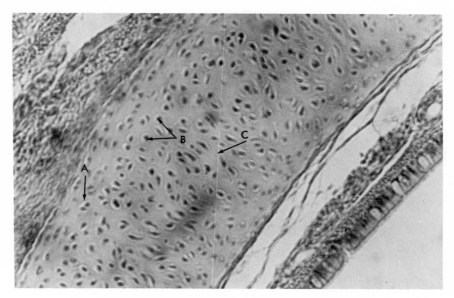

Fig. 1-11. Hyaline cartilage. (✕100.) *A*, Lacuna, *B*, chondrocytes, *C*, matrix.

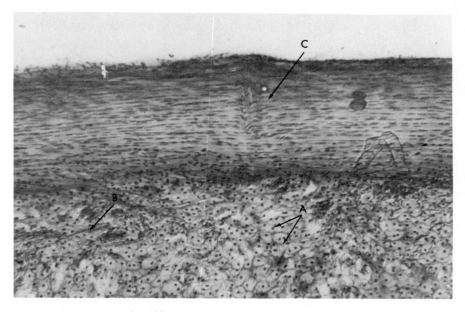

Fig. 1-12. Fibrocartilage. (✕100.) *A*, Small chondrocytes in lacunae, *B*, collagenous fibers in matrix, *C*, dense fibrous connective tissue sheath.

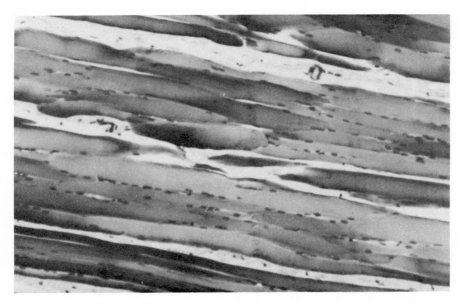

Fig. 1-13. Striated (skeletal, voluntary) muscle. (X100.)

in the body are: skeletal muscle (striated, voluntary), cardiac muscle, and smooth muscle (nonstriated, visceral, involuntary).

The cytoplasm and plasma membrane of these contractile and highly specialized cells are called *sarcoplasm* and *sarcolemma,* respectively. Threadlike *myofibrils* made up of the contractile proteins, *actin and myosin* (the so-called sliding filaments), are found in the sarcoplasm. They are the functional components of muscle cells.

Skeletal muscle composes the mass of muscle organs associated with the skeleton. The cells are long, cylindrical, and multinucleated. The prominent cross-striations, or stripes (Fig. 1-13) seen in these muscle fibers are actually alternate light and dark bands that reflect the arrangement of the contractile proteins in the myofibrils. Each skeletal muscle fiber is innervated by the terminal branch of a motor nerve axon; the junction of nerve and muscle is called the *neuromuscular* or *myoneural* junction. Skeletal muscle is voluntary; that is, it is controlled by the conscious motor areas of the brain.

Cardiac muscle (Fig. 1-14) is found only in the heart muscle, or myocardium. The cells are elongated, branching, and striated. At the junctions between adjacent cells, dark transverse lines, called intercalated disks, can be seen. Each cell has one or more centrally located nuclei. Cardiac muscle, which is involuntary, can contract automatically and rhythmically in the absence of any nervous stimulation. The rate of contraction is, however, controlled in the body by the autonomic nervous system. The impulse for contraction of the whole of the myocardium is normally initiated and transmitted by specialized cardiac muscle cells known as *Purkinje fibers* (Fig. 1-15).

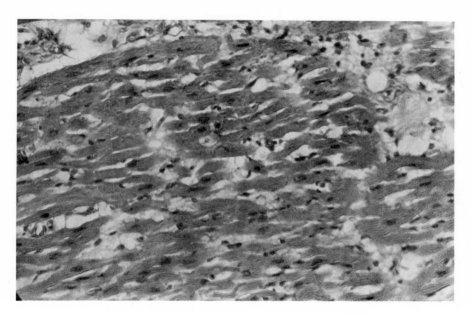

Fig. 1-14. Cardiac muscle fibers (myocardium). (X100.)

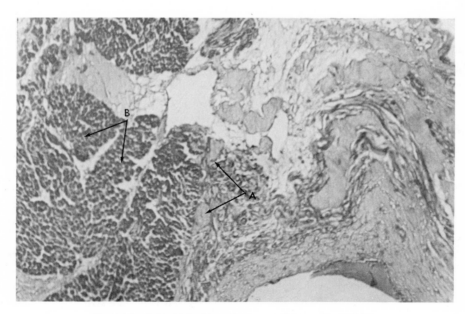

Fig. 1-15. *A*, Purkinje fibers, *B*, myocardial muscle. (X100.)

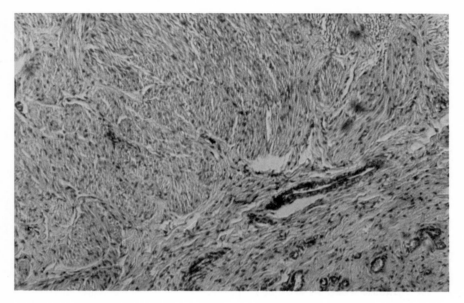

Fig. 1-16. Smooth (visceral, involuntary) muscle fibers. (X100.)

These fibers are found in the sinoatrial and atrioventricular nodes of the right atrium, and they also form an extensive network beneath the endocardium and in the interventricular septum. Purkinje fibers are larger, paler staining, and contain fewer myofibrils than ordinary cardiac muscle cells.

Smooth muscle cells (Fig. 1-16) are involuntary and lack the striations of skeletal and cardiac muscle. The fibers are long, narrow, and tapered at the ends, that is, spindle shaped (fusiform). A single nucleus is found in the wider central portion of the cell. Smooth muscle, also known as visceral muscle, is abundantly distributed in the walls of the hollow organs of the body and in blood and lymphatic vessels.

NERVOUS TISSUE

Nerve cells, like muscle cells, are elongated irritable cells. Their main function is to conduct nervous impulses from one area of the body to another. The nervous system comprises the brain, the spinal cord, and the extensive networks and sensory receptors of the peripheral nerves. The complex structural and functional properties of the nervous system are the province of the specialized fields of macroscopic and microscopic neuroanatomy and neurophysiology.

The cellular unit of the nervous system is a unique cell, the *neuron* (Figs. 1-17 and 1-18). Neurons vary considerably in size and shape, but all are characterized by a rather large cell body, or *perikaryon,* and one or more elongated cytoplasmic processes. In some instances, the end of the cell process may be a foot or more away from the cell body. Neuronal cell bodies are generally found in *nuclei* within the

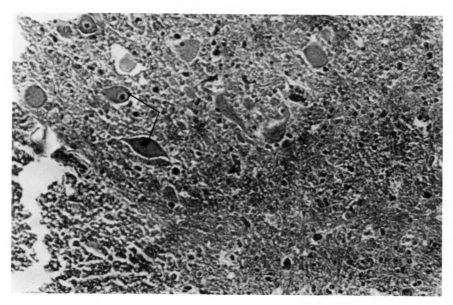

Fig. 1-17. Ganglion cells (neurons) indicated by arrows. (X100.)

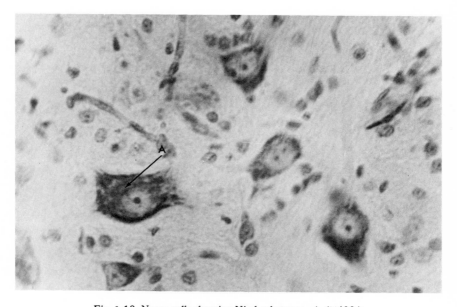

Fig. 1-18. Nerve cells showing Nissl substance, *A.* (X400.)

central nervous system and in *ganglia* outside the central nervous system. The cell bodies of neurons contain *neurofibrils,* a conspicuous *Golgi apparatus,* a rough endoplasmic reticulum studded with ribosomes, which is termed *Nissl substance,* and a single large centrally placed nucleus with one or two prominent nucleoli. The cytoplasmic processes of neurons are *axons,* or axis cylinders, and *dendrites.* The axon is a single process present in all neurons; it is generally referred to as the *nerve fiber.* Most neurons are *multipolar;* that is, they have more than one dendrite. The exceptions are the *unipolar* sensory neurons, with a single-cell process that divides into two outside the cell body, and the *bipolar* neurons of the retina, olfactory mucosa, and inner ear, which have two-cell processes, a dendrite, and an axon. The cell processes of neurons are physiologically distinguished by the fact that dendrites conduct impulses *toward* the cell body, whereas axons conduct *away* from the cell body. Axons vary in diameter, length, and structure.

A unique characteristic of all neurons is the presence of accessory supporting and protective cells of neural origin around cell bodies, dendrites, and axons. In the peripheral nervous system, axons are wrapped around by *Schwann cells,* which form the *neurilemma,* an investing sheath. A lipid substance, myelin, is a component of the plasma membrane of Schwann cells. If the axon is wrapped extensively in a spiral pattern by its Schwann cells, it is said to be *myelinated.* If the wrapping is not extensive, or only partial, the fiber is *nonmyelinated.* In myelinated fibers, the junction of two Schwann cells appears as an indentation called the *node of Ranvier.* A neurilemma is essential for the regeneration of the axon. Axons in the central nervous system, which lack the Schwann cell neurilemma, are generally incapable of regeneration. The cell bodies of neurons in the ganglia outside the central nervous system are surrounded by small flat cells called *satellite cells,* which are similar to Schwann cells. Within the central nervous system, the supporting and protective functions of the Schwann cells and satellite cells are carried out by *neuroglia* (Gr. *glia,* glue). The glial cells that form the sheath and myelin of axons in the brain and the spinal cord are called *oligodendroglia* or *oligodendrocytes.* They are also found in association with cell bodies of neurons in the central nervous system in a manner similar to the satellite cells of ganglia. Another type of glial cell found in the central nervous system is the *astrocyte,* a cell with many branched processes. These cells are interposed between capillaries and neuron cell bodies. Astrocytes are believed to control the diffusion of substances from the bloodstream into the tissue spaces of the central nervous system, and thus constitute what is known as the blood-brain barrier. A third cell type classified as glia is the *microglia,* although these cells are not of neural (ectodermal) origin. Microglia are small mobile phagocytes of the central nervous system. They are particularly active during injury and infection.

2

Histologic design of organs

The study of cells is called *cytology,* and the study of tissues is called *histology.* The study of microscopic architecture of organs is called microscopic anatomy or special histology.

All the body tissues and organs arise from the differentiation of the three primary germ layers of the embryo, the *ectoderm* (outer skin), *mesoderm* (middle skin), and *entoderm* (inner skin). During embryologic development, part of the ectoderm forms the neural tube from which nerve tissue arises, and the remainder forms the epithelium of the integument and the oral cavity. The entoderm forms the epithelial lining and the glands of the alimentary and respiratory tracts. The mesoderm forms the epithelium of the urinary and genital systems and two additional specialized forms of epithelium, the mesothelium of the serous membranes and the endothelium, which lines blood and lymph vessels and the heart. The rest of the mesoderm forms striated, cardiac, and smooth muscle and also differentiates into *mesenchyme,* the embryonic connective tissue from which the various types of connective tissue, including cartilage, bone, and blood, evolve.

It will be apparent to anyone viewing a section of an organ under a microscope that not only is there marked structural variation among cells of different tissues, but there is an equal amount of variation in the pattern of distribution of tissues within organs. The spatial arrangements of the tissue components that make up an organ are generally unique to that organ and are closely correlated with its functions.

Some organ systems of the body are made up predominantly of one type of tissue, for example, the central and peripheral nervous systems, the (voluntary) muscular system, and the skeletal system. Others are more complex structurally and contain a variety of tissues. In general, certain architectural features of organs are characteristic and can be listed as follows:

1. The apposition, particularly in solid organs, of tissues that are primarily involved in the function of the organ (the *parenchyma*), and the supportive tissues making up the framework of the organ (the *stroma*)
2. The presence of an outer connective tissue covering, or *capsule,* in most organs
3. The association of nonvascular epithelial linings with a subepithelial vascular

connective tissue lamina (layer); in areas where the epithelium is greatly stratified, the lamina is often thrown up into ridges *(papillae)* that increase the area of contact between the two tissues

4. The presence in some solid organs of two structurally and often functionally distinct zones—an outer shell, or *cortex,* and an inner core, or *medulla*

5. The arrangement of several different layers *(tunics)* in the walls of hollow organs lined by moist mucous membranes; although these show some individual variations, the general pattern from the *lumen* to the outer covering is *mucosa* (epithelium, connective tissue lamina, occasionally smooth muscle), *submucosa* (connective tissue), *muscularis* (smooth or striated muscle), and *adventitia* (fibrous connective tissue), or *serosa* (mesothelium)

6. The structural plan of the walls of blood and lymphatic vessels; the innermost *tunica intima* (endothelium, connective tissue), the middle *tunica media* (smooth muscle, connective tissue), and the outer *tunica adventitia* (connective tissue), all of which gradually thin out as the vessels become smaller until in the capillaries only the endothelial lining is left

Of the four primary tissues, epithelium probably forms the most highly specialized and widely distributed structures. Practically all the secreting surface membranes (mucous and serous) and the secreting glands (endocrine and exocrine) of the body are composed of epithelium. These structures may be a relatively minor feature of an organ or, as in the case of predominantly secretory organs, they may compose the entire parenchyma.

SEROUS AND MUCOUS MEMBRANES

The body cavities are lined with *serous membranes,* known as the *pleurae* (in the thorax), *pericardium* (around the heart), and *peritoneum* (in the abdomen). In each instance, a portion lines the cavity (parietal portion) and a portion is reflected over the organs, or viscera, contained in the cavity (visceral portion). The surface of all the serous membranes is covered by mesothelium, a specialized simple squamous epithelium that is derived from embryonic mesoderm. A similar epithelium lines the subdural and subarachnoid spaces of the central nervous system. The mesothelium rests on a loose connective tissue lamina, beneath which there may be an additional connective tissue layer, the subserosa. The serous membranes secrete a small amount of clear serous fluid, which usually contains desquamated mesothelial cells, macrophages, and leukocytes. An increase in the volume of this fluid may occur in inflammatory conditions and malignant diseases. The tunica serosa, an outer coat of the wall of some hollow organs, is part of the visceral serous membrane of the cavity in which the organ is located.

The *mucous membranes* line the hollow organs and passageways of the body. They consist of various types of surface epithelium, simple or stratified, a connective tissue lamina with or without smooth muscle, and a fibrous submucosa. They are characterized in most instances by mucus-secreting epithelial cells or glands that lubricate the luminal surface with a slimy viscous material.

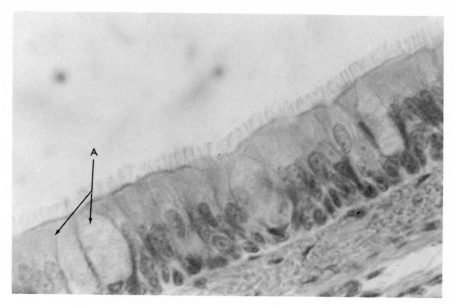

Fig. 2-1. Unicellular mucous glands. *A*, Goblet cells; note ciliated border. (X1000.)

ENDOCRINE AND EXOCRINE GLANDS

Endocrine glands secrete substances *(hormones)* directly into the bloodstream, and *exocrine glands* secrete substances, usually by way of ducts, onto an epithelial surface. Both types of glands originate from the invagination (infolding or pushing in) of an epithelial sheet during the development of the embryo. The exocrine glands permanently retain their connection with the surface. The endocrine glands are cut off from the surface and, in most cases, no longer resemble the epithelium from which they arose. The architecture of endocrine glands shows much individual variation but, in general, cells are arranged in compact groups surrounded by rich vascular networks and connective tissue stroma. Some of the glands of the body, for example, the liver, pancreas, and the gonads, contain both endocrine and exocrine components. Endocrine glands are described in subsequent chapters.

Exocrine glands are classified in several ways: by the type of secretion, by the manner in which the secretion is released, and by the microscopic arrangement of the cellular units of the gland. A variety of products are synthesized and secreted, including sex cells (ova and spermatozoa), sweat, milk, sebum, cerumen, mucus, and serous substances containing enzymes. *Holocrine* glands secrete living or degenerated cells (sex glands and sebaceous glands, respectively); *apocrine* glands are an intermediate form that secrete pinched-off top portions of cytoplasm (mammary glands); *merocrine* glands discharge secretion from intact cells. Merocrine glands include the largest group of secreting glands in the body, the mucous and serous glands. The simplest (unicellular) mucus-secreting merocrine gland is the goblet cell

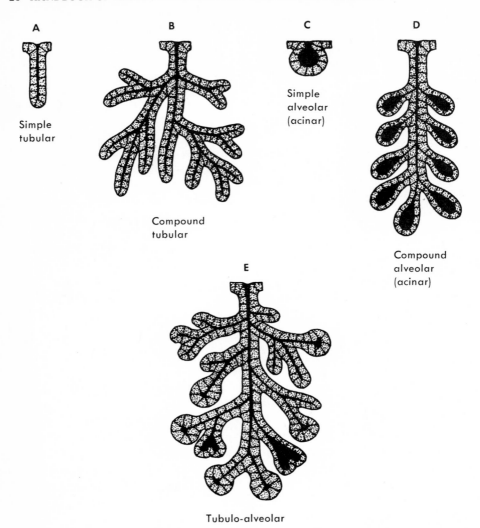

A

Simple
tubular

B

Compound
tubular

C

Simple
alveolar
(acinar)

D

Compound
alveolar
(acinar)

E

Tubulo-alveolar

Fig. 2-2. Diagram of multicellular glands. (From Phillips; J. B.: Development of vertebrate anatomy, St. Louis, 1975, The C. V. Mosby Co.)

found in intestinal and respiratory tract epithelium (Fig. 2-1). More complex mucous glands, serous glands, and mixed seromucous glands are found mainly in the digestive tract. Mucus is a thick protein-polysaccharide compound, which may be washed out during routine histologic processing of tissues. As a result, the mucous cells in a gland are usually pale staining. Serous cells secrete a clear albuminous substance often containing enzymes. These cells are basophilic and generally dark staining. In a gland with mixed seromucous elements, such as the submandibular (salivary) gland, the darker serous cells appear as crescent-shaped caps (demilunes) above the pale mucous cells.

Multicellular glands consist of one or more secreting endpieces and either single or branching ducts leading to a surface. *Simple* glands have a single duct; *compound* glands have a branching system of ducts exiting from a variable number of secreting endpieces. The arrangement of the secreting epithelium in the endpieces is also used to classify the gland. Endpieces in human exocrine glands are commonly either cylindrical in shape *(tubular glands)*, spherical or pear shaped *(alveolar* or *acinar glands)*, or a combination of both *(tubuloalveolar glands)*. Diagrams of simple and compound multicellular glands are shown in Fig. 2-2. However, the arrangement of endpieces and ducts, as shown in the diagram, is not usually seen in routine histologic sections. Exocrine glands in cross section characteristically appear as clusters of small spherical cavities enclosed by a rim of epithelial cells and surrounded by connective tissue.

3

Abnormal tissues—tumors

The production of new cells in the body by mitosis in normally a controlled and orderly process that is adjusted to the needs of the body, that is, the replacement of cells lost through injury or aging and the growth of body structures in a young developing organism. When one or more cells in a tissue start to reproduce excessively, an abnormal mass or tissue, or *tumor* or *neoplasm* (new growth), results. The change (mutation) in the original cell or cells that started the tumor is transmitted to their descendants, so that all the generations of cells that follow inherit the tendency to uncontrolled growth.

Tumors may be *benign* (noncancerous) or *malignant* (cancerous). Benign tumors are generally localized orderly overgrowths of tissue, enclosed in a capsule or connective tissue sheath. The cells of a benign tumor usually closely resemble the normal cells from which they arose. Mitotic figures may or may not be present, depending on the growth rate of the tumor. The presence of dividing cells is not, in itself, a proof of malignancy. Provided that there is an adequate blood supply, benign tumors are capable of continued growth and may become quite large. However, the cells do not *metastasize* (spread to distant parts of the body). The symptoms usually caused by these growths are due to obstruction or interference with the normal functions of adjacent organs. In addition, benign tumors in endocrine glands may produce an excessive amount of hormones. Although it is a common belief that every benign tumor is potentially cancerous, there is no conclusive evidence to indicate that these cells have any greater tendency to undergo malignant transformation than normal cells.

The term cancer includes all malignant tumors, regardless of the tissue in which they originated. Malignancy is characterized primarily by a disorganization, or even disappearance, of the typical histologic pattern or architecture of a tissue. This condition is known as *anaplasia*, meaning the loss of normal differentiation or organization. The degree of anaplasia in the many different types of cancer varies considerably. Some tumors appear to be so well differentiated that it may be difficult to distinguish them from benign growths; others may be so undifferentiated, or anaplastic, that it may be difficult to identify the tissue of origin. Most malignant tumors fall somewhere between these two extremes. As a rule, the more malignant tumors are more anaplastic. Besides the overall structural disorder, individual cancer cells within the tumor may show much variation in size and shape *(pleomorphism)*. Thus it is not unusual to find atypical and bizarre cells that bear little or no resemblance to their neighbors.

Growth of malignant tumors may be rapid or slow, with many or few mitotic figures present. In general, malignant tumors grow more rapidly and show more mitotic figures than benign tumors. The presence of abnormal or asymmetric mitoses almost always indicates malignancy.

Malignant tumors are usually not encapsulated, and grow by infiltration. A typical microscopic picture is one showing columns of cancer cells invading the surrounding normal tissues. The demands of the ever-increasing cell mass for a blood supply to nourish it and carry away its waste products are enormous, and recent research indicates that malignant tumors secrete a substance that stimulates the growth of new blood vessels. By whatever mechanism, malignant tumors are able to compete successfully for the available blood supply, the end results being the destruction of the normal tissue along the path of invasion and its replacement by neoplastic cells. Not all tissues are equally susceptible to malignant invasion. The fibrous capsules of viscera, such as the liver, kidney, and spleen, the periosteum of bone, ligaments, tendons, and cartilage, and the fibroelastic tunics of arteries resist neoplastic infiltration.

The stroma (supporting framework) of malignant tumors may consist of varying amounts of fibrous connective tissue, lymphocytes, plasma cells, neutrophils, eosinophils, and tissue macrophages. The stroma is not cancerous, and is derived from the connective tissues of the surrounding normal structures and the wandering leukocytes of the body. In some cancers, particularly the so-called *scirrhous* (hard) types, there is an overgrowth of dense fibrous tissue around small isolated islands of tumor cells. Many tumors also show collections of leukocytes and macrophages, which appear to be attracted by the presence of necrotic (dead) cells and the liberation of metabolites (by-products of tumor metabolism) in the vicinity.

METASTASIS

One of the most characteristic features of malignant tumors is their tendency to metastasize, that is, to produce secondary growths in other parts of the body. Metastasis of tumors is defined as the transfer of malignant cells from one part (a primary focus) to distant parts (secondary foci). The cells are conveyed by blood vessels and lymphatics. Metastases are the direct result of local tumor infiltration of thin-walled lymphatic vessels and veins; arteries and arterioles are rarely invaded. The tumor grows through the vessel wall, proliferates in the lumen, and may even extend in a continous column along the lumina of larger vessels. Malignant cells do not adhere to each other as strongly as normal tissue cells do. Once inside a vessel, microscopic clumps *(emboli)* of tumor cells tend to detach from the main mass and are carried along by the lymph flow to regional lymph nodes or by the venous blood flow to other organs. Not all tumor emboli are equally successful in implanting and growing in distant foci, but where large numbers of malignant cells are shed into the blood and lymph, metastatic growth of a small proportion of them is inevitable.

Histologically, metastatic growths almost always closely resemble the original primary tumor.

Lymph node metastases

Detached tumor emboli are carried to lymph nodes by the lymph flow. This mode of spread is common in tumors of the stomach, intestine, breast, uterus, and lung. The emboli grow in the node until the entire structure is replaced by neoplastic tissue (Fig. 3-1). Lymph node metastases are often a source for further spread of the tumor, by lymphatic channels draining the invaded node.

Skeletal metastases

The skeleton is one of the more frequent sites of metastatic growth (Fig. 3-2). Tumor emboli reach bone by spreading through veins. The bones most commonly affected are those containing red marrow, such as the vertebrae, ribs, skull, femur, and pelvis. The tumor growth is generally *osteolytic* (dissolving the bony matrix) and, by invasion of the bone marrow, interferes with normal *hemopoiesis* (blood cell production by marrow cells). Thus, these metastases often cause pathologic fractures of bone, as well as severe anemia.

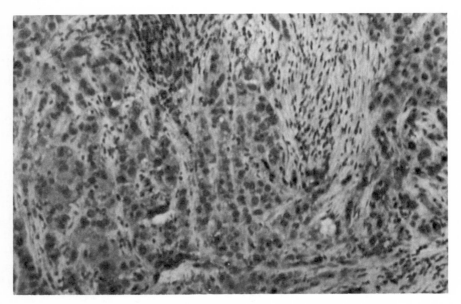

Fig. 3-1. Metastatic carcinoma in lymph node. Masses of cells with atypical nuclei have invaded the node, replacing normal nodal tissue. Fibrous stroma at upper right. (X100.)

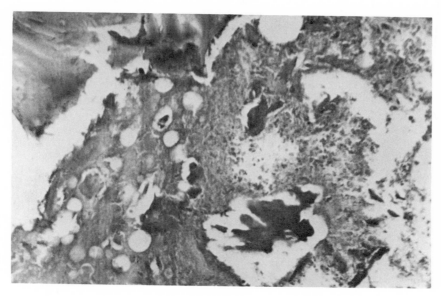

Fig. 3-2 Metastatic tumor in bone. Normal bone matrix is destroyed. Necrotic (dead) tissue in center. (×100.)

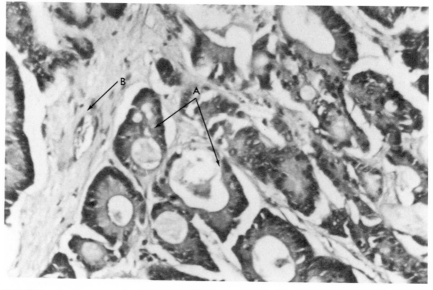

Fig. 3-3. Liver metastases. *A*, Columnar cell adenocarcinoma, *B* loose fibrous stroma. Normal liver parenchyma absent. (×100.)

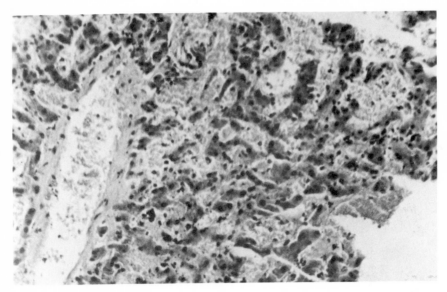

Fig. 3-4. Metastatic carcinoma in lung tissue. Cords of dark-staining malignant epithelial cells have replaced lung tissue and are infiltrating blood vessel on the left. (×100.)

Metastases to the liver and the lungs

Two vital organs, the liver and the lungs, are the most frequent sites of blood-borne metastases. Tumor emboli reach the liver (Fig. 3-3) by way of the portal vein and its tributaries, and the lung (Fig. 3-4) by way of the venous return to the right side of the heart.

In the liver, tumor cells extend along the capillary spaces between the cords of hepatic cells and grow uniformly into the surrounding tissue, penetrating the hepatic veins and destroying the normal liver structures. Because of its rich vascular supply, the liver provides a favorable medium for growth, and tumor cells proliferate rapidly in this organ.

Metastatic growth in the lungs is usually multiple and bilateral. The tumors replace the normal lung architecture and use the spongy network of alveoli as a stroma.

NOMENCLATURE OF TUMORS

There are many specific names for tumors, but certain general rules can be followed. Most terms for tumors, benign and malignant, have the suffix *-oma* (Gr. *oma*, swelling), meaning a tumor or neoplasm. The first part of the name usually indicates the tissue of origin: thus, *lipoma* (a tumor of fatty tissue), *fibroma* (a tumor of fibrous connective tissue), *lymphoma* (a tumor of lymphoid tissue), and *glioma* (a tumor of neuroglial tissue). The foregoing names generally indicate benign growths. Malignant tumors are classified mainly as *carcinomas* (cancer arising from epithelial tissues) and *sarcomas* (cancers originating from connective tissue elements). Carcinomas and sarcomas are further subgrouped to indicate specifically the tissue of origin: thus, *adenocarcinoma* (Gr. *aden,* gland; carcinoma of glandular epithelium), *osteosarcoma* (malignant tumor of bone), *liposarcoma* (malignant tumor of adipose tissue), *lymphosarcoma* (malignant tumor of lymphoid tissue), and *melanosarcoma,* or *melanoma* (malignancy involving the melanin-producing cells of the body). Malignant tumors composed of white blood cells (leukocytes) are usually classified as *leukemias.*

4

The integument

The integument of the body includes the skin and cutaneous appendages such as nails, hair, and sebaceous and sweat glands. Integumentary structures in animals other than man include feathers, claws, scales, and horns.

An intact skin protects the body against bacterial invasion from the outside, prevents loss of fluids from the interior of the body, helps to maintain body temperature, and contains various nerve receptors for cold, heat, pain, touch, and pressure.

Skin consists of an *epidermis* and a *dermis*. The epidermis is composed of keratinized stratified squamous epithelium. It varies in thickness from 0.07 to 1.4 mm. It is thinnest in the eyelids and thickest in the soles of the feet (plantar skin) and palms of the hands (palmar skin). The epidermis, like other epithelium, has no blood supply of its own and is dependent on the vascular connective tissue bed below it for nourishment and removal of waste products. There may be as many as five layers, or strata, in the epidermis. These are, from the deepest to the surface strata: stratum germinativum (germinating layer), stratum spinosum (spiny layer), stratum granulosum (granular layer), stratum lucidum (clear layer), and stratum corneum (horny or cornified layer). In thin skin (Fig. 4-1), the stratum germinativum and stratum corneum are usually the only layers that can be distinguished. In thick skin, all five layers may be present.

All stratified epithelium is characterized by a continuous loss (sloughing off) of dead cells from the surface layers; these cells are replaced by the proliferation of the cells of the deepest layer. In the epidermis, the proliferating, or *germinative,* layer (also called the basal layer) is a single layer of modified, darkly staining (basophilic) columnar cells with large nuclei. These cells receive most of the diffused nutrients from the connective tissue dermis that lies immediately below them. Basal cells are mitotically active. Above them are several layers of polyhedral (many-sided) cells that are interconnected by microscopic bridges, or spines, thus accounting for the term *stratum spinosum.* The *stratum granulosum* varies in thickness. The flattened cells of this layer contain the first granules of *keratin,* an insoluble fibrous sulfur-containing protein that waterproofs the skin. Keratin is present in large amounts in hair, nails,

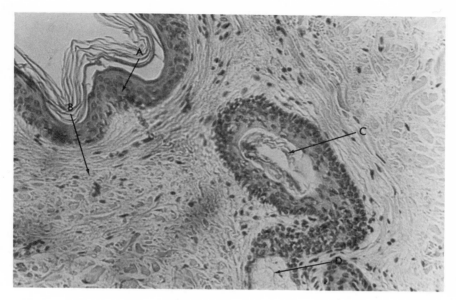

Fig. 4-1. Thin skin. *A*, Epidermis, *B*, dermis, *C*, hair follicle, *D*, sebaceous gland. (×100.)

horny tissue such as callus, and in tooth enamel. In some areas the *stratum lucidum,* a thin clear layer of flattened, closely packed cells lacking nuclei, is interposed between the granular layer and the topmost *stratum corneum*. The outermost layers of epithelium are composed of dried, flattened cells that have lost their nuclei. The cytoplasm of the cells of this stratum corneum is completely replaced by keratin.

Mingling with the cells of the basal layer is a group of specialized nonepithelial elements called *melanocytes*. These cells manufacture the pigment, melanin, which is responsible for skin color. The pigment is transferred by melanocytes to adjoining epidermal cells. In individuals with light-colored skin, the pigment is limited to the basal layer. In dark-skinned people, melanin is found throughout the stratum germinativum and in the stratum granulosum.

Underlying the stratum germinativum is a compact layer of dense connective tissue called the *dermis,* or *corium*. It extends from the epidermis to the subcutaneous areolar and fat tissue. The dermis contains the blood vessels, lymphatics, nerves and nerve endings, glands, and other specialized cutaneous structures of the skin. The upper portion of the dermis that is in contact with the basal layer of the epidermis is thrown up into elevations or ridges called the *dermal papillae*. These ridges are especially prominent in palmar and plantar skin.

Associated with the integument are various cutaneous appendages, such as cutaneous glands (sebaceous, sweat, and ceruminous glands), hair, and nails. These structures are all histologically derived from epidermal epithelium.

Sebaceous glands (Fig. 4-2) are found everywhere in the skin, with the exception

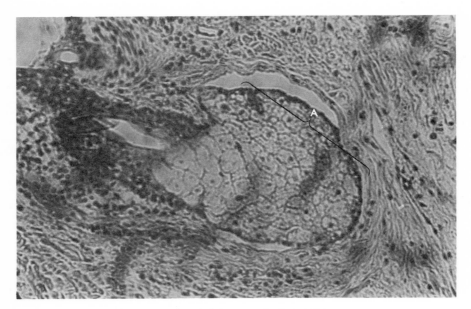

Fig. 4-2. *A*, Sebaceous gland. (X100.)

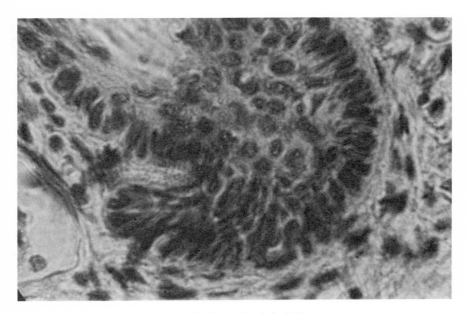

Fig. 4-3. Sweat gland. (X400.)

of palmar and plantar skin. They lie in the dermis and produce a lipid secretion called *sebum,* which usually passes through a duct into a hair follicle. Sebum lubricates the hair and the skin.

Sweat glands (Fig. 4-3) are located in the dermis of most of the skin in the body. They are coiled tubular glands that empty through ducts directly onto the skin surface. Sweat glands regulate the body temperature by the cooling effect of water evaporation from the surface of the skin. Sweat also contains urea and salts.

Ceruminous glands resemble large sweat glands. They are found only in the skin of the external auditory canal. They secrete a protective waxy substance called *cerumen.*

Mammary glands (milk-secreting glands) are also examples of modified sweat glands.

Hairs are hardened, keratinized epithelial structures. A hair follicle has an inner layer, which is a continuation of the epidermis, and an outer connective tissue covering. The pigment in hair is melanin. Associated with hair follicles are bands of smooth muscle, called *arrector pili* muscles, and one or more sebaceous glands.

Nails are outgrowths of epidermal cells that have become filled with hard keratin. The dermis underlying these cells is modified to form the nail bed.

TUMORS OF THE SKIN

Two malignant tumors that can occur in the skin are illustrated. The first is a squamous carcinoma of the skin (a cancer arising from the stratified squamous

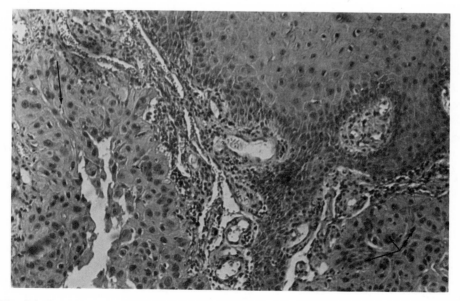

Fig. 4-4. Squamous carcinoma of the skin; malignant cells indicated by arrows. Nuclei show marked variation in size and shape. (X100.)

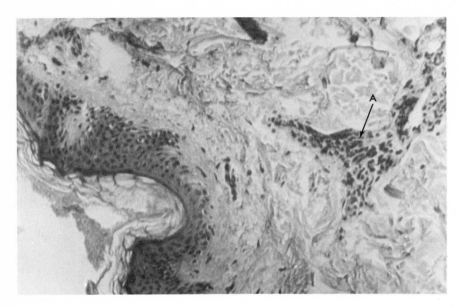

Fig. 4-5. Malignant melanoma of the skin. *A*, Mass of pigmented melanoma cells infiltrating dermis. (X100.)

epithelium of the epidermis) (Fig. 4-4). This tumor is formed when a group of epidermal cells begins to proliferate (increase in number) in an uncontrolled manner. The cells appear atypical, displaying marked differences in size and shape (pleomorphism). The nuclei are large in comparison with the cytoplasm. Many mitotic figures can be seen. As these cells increase in number, they disrupt the normal architecture of the skin. Fingerlike columns of malignant epithelial cells break through the basal layer of the epidermis and penetrate into the corium, from which they spread out in all directions. Frequently, the cells of a squamous carcinoma appear to be arranging themselves into more or less normal epidermal layers; certain areas of the tumor may resemble the stratum germinativum; others, the stratum spinosum and stratum corneum. Some cancer cells may even produce keratin like their normal counterparts. This process is known as *differentiation*. When a tumor shows evidence of differentiation, it is considered to be less malignant and more curable than a tumor mass that is completely disorganized (anaplastic) and bears no resemblance to any normal tissue structures.

Fig. 4-5 shows a malignant melanoma (or melanosarcoma). This tumor can start in the skin or in other organs. The tumor cells are not of epithelial origin, but are derived from melanocytes. Normal melanocytes are nonepithelial, star-shaped cells that can be found scattered among the basal cells of the epidermis. They produce the black pigment of the skin, melanin, which is then picked up by the cells of the stratum germinativum.

Many melanomas arise from a special type of mole (pigmented spot) on the skin, which is called a junctional nevus. The nevus, a cluster of melanocytes found at the borderline (junction) of the epidermis and the dermis, is itself benign. However, the cells of a nevus of this type can undergo sudden malignant change. The cells and their nuclei enlarge, many abnormal mitotic figures are evident, and there is a rapid invasion of the underlying dermis and of the blood vessels and lymphatic vessels in the dermis (metastasis). The melanoma shown is pigmented (the cells contain melanin granules). However, some of these tumors contain no pigment and are difficult to diagnose.

5

Bone and bone marrow

The human skeleton is composed of 206 bones, which have a thin, hard *(compact)*, bony layer on the outside and spongy *(cancellous)* bone tissue on the inside. The long bones of the body contain a central *marrow* cavity, bordered by spongy bone; in other bones, the interior consists only of spongy bone. Bone marrow occupies the marrow cavities and the interspaces of spongy bone. The *periosteum,* a tough fibrous connective tissue sheath, covers the outer surfaces of bones, except for the joint (articular) surfaces, which are lined with hyaline cartilage.

THE CELLS AND MATRIX OF BONE

Bone is made up of a rigid matrix in which are scattered bone cells *(osteocytes)* enclosed in tiny cavities *(lacunae)*. Cells immobilized in lacunae are characteristic of semirigid and rigid connective tissues, that is, cartilage and bone. Osteocytes have a granular *basophilic* cytoplasm and a large oval nucleus. They are the mature forms of *osteoblasts* (the more primitive osteogenic cells), which synthesize the bony matrix. The cell bodies of osteocytes contain many fine cytoplasmic processes, which radiate outward and contact the processes of neighboring cells. The processes lie in minute channels *(canaliculi)* in the bony matrix and can be seen as a series of lines or dots connecting each lacuna.

Another type of bone cell, often seen where parts of the bone are being resorbed or dissolved, is a giant multinucleate cell called the *osteoclast* (bone destroyer). These cells are active during bone growth, enlarging the marrow cavities and facilitating the increase in the dimensions of bones.

The matrix of bone is made up of an organic framework of dense collagen fibers embedded in a mucoid cement, and a mineral component consisting mainly of salts of calcium phosphate. The calcium salts are deposited on the organic matrix; both components of the matrix are synthesized and secreted mainly by osteoblasts. The organic material forms 30% to 40% of bone substance, and the mineral salts form 60% to 70%. The calcium content of the matrix, particularly that of spongy bone, serves as a reservoir for the maintenance of blood calcium levels. Calcium is released from bone by the action of the parathyroid hormone. Its release is inhibited by the action of calcitonin from the thyroid gland. The antagonistic action of the two hormones constitutes a feedback mechanism that regulates calcium balance in the body. In old age, the mineral component is often increased, causing bones to become relatively brittle. In rickets, the mineral component is decreased, leaving the bones softer and more pliable.

STRUCTURE OF COMPACT AND CANCELLOUS BONE

Bone matrix is characteristically laid down in *lamellae* (thin plates). In compact bone the lamellae are regularly arranged in concentric rings, which are a microscopic counterpart of the annual growth rings found in cross sections of tree trunks. Each set of concentric lamellae, containing from four to twenty separate plates, constitutes a *haversian system,* the histologic structural unit of compact bone (Figs. 5-1 and 5-2). In the center of each haversian system is a haversian canal containing blood vessels, unmyelinated nerves, and lymphatic capillaries. The central canals communicate with the periosteum and the marrow spaces via Volkmann's canals, which run at right angles to them. Osteocytes in lacunae are interspersed at regular intervals along the concentric plates. Numerous radiating canaliculi connect the lacunae to each other and to the central canal. The arrangement is such that, despite the rigid matrix, nutrients and waste materials can be exchanged between the osteocytes and the blood.

Macroscopically, spongy bone has a honeycomb appearance; microscopically, the lamellae may be arranged in irregular plates, *trabeculae* (small beams or bars), tubes, or

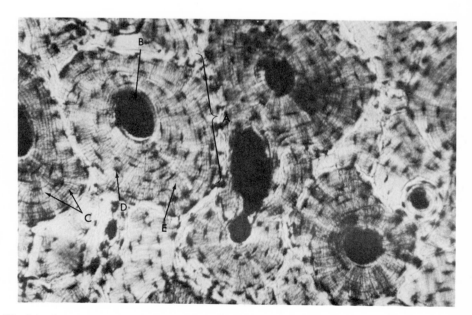

Fig. 5-1. Compact bone. (×100.) *A*, Haversian system, *B*, haversian canal, *C*, lamellae, *D*, osteocyte in lacuna, *E*, canaliculi.

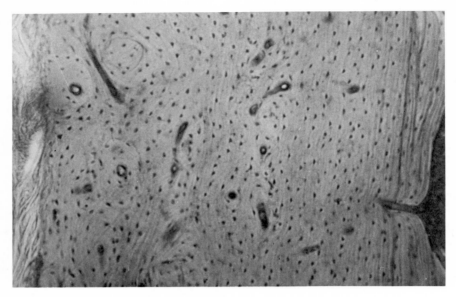

Fig. 5-2. Decalcified bone. (×100.)

hollow globes. The characteristic haversian system is absent, although some areas of spongy bone may show concentric lamellae.

BONE FORMATION (OSTEOGENESIS)

With the exception of the flat cranial bones and some facial bones, the skeleton of the developing fetus consists of hyaline cartilage models of future bones. Early in fetal life, areas in the cartilage matrix become calcified, and the chondrocytes (cartilage cells) in these locations degenerate and die. At the same time, bone-forming osteoblasts differentiate from the *perichondrium* (connective tissue sheath around cartilage) (Fig. 5-3) and deposit a matrix of ground substance and collagenous fibers, called *osteoid,* which is subsequently reinforced with calcium salts. The first bony trabeculae appear as irregular masses in the osteoid substance. These primary centers of ossification are the only bone areas present in the cartilage skeleton of the fetus. After birth, secondary ossification centers appear. Spongy bone is formed before compact bone. The replacement of cartilage by bone is known as *intracartilaginous,* or *endochondral, bone development.* The histologic picture of bone formation from cartilage shows rather straight rows of lacunae containing chondrocytes, which appear more and more swollen and degenerated as they near the advancing zone of newly formed bone.

In the flat bones of the skull and the face, bone is formed from a primitive mesenchymal connective tissue membrane. Osteoblasts arise from this tissue and form centers of ossification within the membrane, laying down osteoid and then calcium

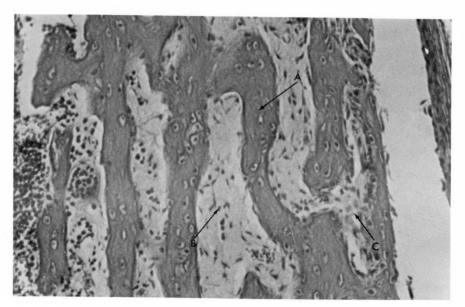

Fig. 5-3. Formation of bone. *A*, Bone matrix with osteocytes, *B*, osteogenic connective tissue, *C*, osteoblasts. (×100.)

salts. This type of bone formation is called *intramembranous ossification*. Most of the spongy and compact bone of the cranium is formed during fetal life, but membranous gaps in the cranium, called fontanels, persist for varying periods of time after birth.

BONE MARROW

Bone marrow, a specialized connective tissue, is found in the marrow cavities in the shafts of long bones and in the spaces of spongy bone. Red bone marrow is actively hemopoietic tissue that produces blood cells. Inactive bone marrow consists mainly of fat cells and is termed yellow marrow. During childhood, all bone marrow is red marrow. In the adult, the marrow of the long bones is yellow marrow, and the red marrow is confined to the cranium, vertebrae, ribs, pelvis, and sternum. Yellow marrow can be transformed to active red marrow to meet the needs of the body. The surface of the irregular bony trabeculae that enclose the marrow is covered by a delicate *endosteum,* a membrane composed mainly of osteoblasts.

The stroma of red bone marrow is made up of reticular connective tissue containing both fibers and reticular cells. Within the meshes of reticular fibers are the hemopoietic components of bone marrow, that is, red and white blood cells (erythrocytes and leukocytes) in various stages of maturation. Scattered fat cells are also seen here. Flattened phagocytic reticular cells (macrophages) line an extensive network of sinusoids that runs through the hemopoietic tissue, connecting arterial and

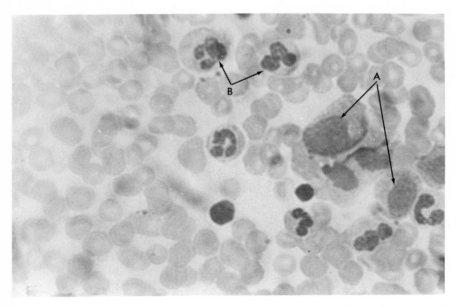

Fig. 5-4. Normal bone marrow. *A*, Myelocytes, *B*, mature polymorphonuclear leukocytes. (×400.)

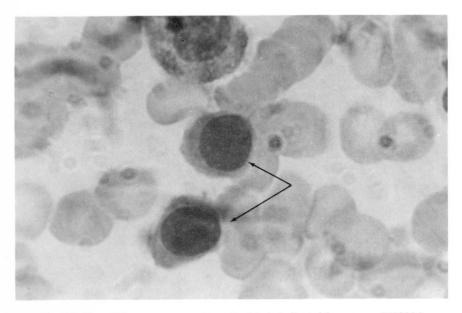

Fig. 5-5. Normal bone marrow; two erythroblasts indicated by arrows. (×1000.)

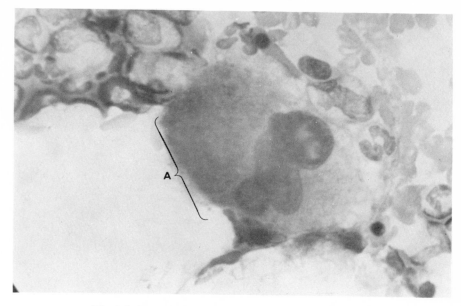

Fig. 5-6. Normal bone marrow. *A*, megakaryocyte. (×400.)

venous vessels. Mature blood cells and platelets produced in the marrow enter the blood stream by infiltrating through the thin walls of the sinusoids.

Of the blood cells seen in hemopoietic marrow (Figs. 5-4 and 5-5), about 65% are immature and mature cells of the granulocytic series. The juvenile forms include myeloblasts, myelocytes, and metamyelocytes; the mature cells are neutrophilic, eosinophilic, and basophilic granulocytes. About 20% are nucleated red blood cells called erythroblasts and normoblasts. Normoblasts eventually lose their nuclei by extrusion and become erythrocytes. Less than 1% are megakaryocytes, large complex cells that form platelets by fragmentation of their abundant cytoplasm (Fig. 5-6). About 10% are lymphocytes, 2% are monocytes, and less than 1% are plasma cells.

Descriptions of the cells that most commonly appear in peripheral blood and lymphoid tissue are included in the next two chapters.

Bone marrow is the site of blood cell production and blood cell differentiation. It supplies the mature blood cells and the platelets of blood. The phagocytes of bone marrow remove damaged and senile blood cells from the circulation. Bone marrow also plays an important part in the immunologic mechanisms of the body.

TUMORS OF BONE AND BONE MARROW
Osteogenic sarcoma (osteosarcoma)

Osteogenic sarcoma is one of the most common primary malignancies of bone (Figs. 5-7 and 5-8). It occurs most frequently in males of a relatively young age group,

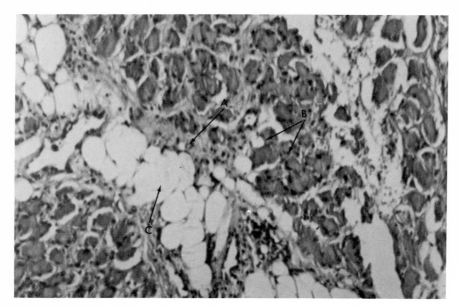

Fig. 5-7. Osteogenic sarcoma. *A*, Small sarcoma cells and deposits of osteoid, *B*, spicules of tumor bone, *C*, tumor infiltrating fatty marrow. (X100.)

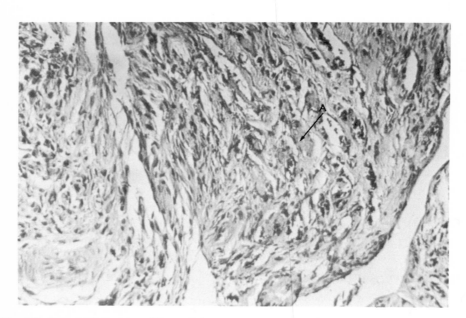

Fig. 5-8. Osteogenic sarcoma. More cellular portion of tumor with sarcomatous spindle cells. *A*, Formation of osteoid. (X100.)

and usually involves the ends of long bones such as the femur, tibia, and humerus. The malignant cells arise from primitive osteoblasts and often appear spindle shaped. These cells invariably produce osteoid and clumps of tumor bone. The matrix is deposited between strands of tumor cells. The histologic appearance of the tumor may vary in different areas. The central portion of the sarcoma may show well-differentiated bone deposits, whereas the advancing borders of the growth may be predominantly composed of spindle-shaped sarcoma cells.

Osteogenic sarcoma tends to invade the marrow cavity and the periosteum. Blood-borne metastases usually occur in the lungs.

It has been demonstrated that osteogenic sarcomas appear after heavy local irradiation of bone by x-rays or gamma rays from radioactive elements such as radium and strontium 85 that are deposited and concentrated in the skeleton. This phenomenon was first observed several decades ago in a group of young women who had ingested radium while painting clock dials with a luminous paint containing this substance. A significant proportion of the group suffered radium poisoning and subsequently developed osteogenic sarcomas.

Multiple myeloma (plasma cell myeloma)

Multiple myeloma (Fig. 5-9) is a relatively rare neoplastic disease, which produces multiple punched-out areas of bone erosion in the ribs, sternum, vertebrae, and skull. In adults, these bones contain red marrow. The malignant cells closely resemble plasma

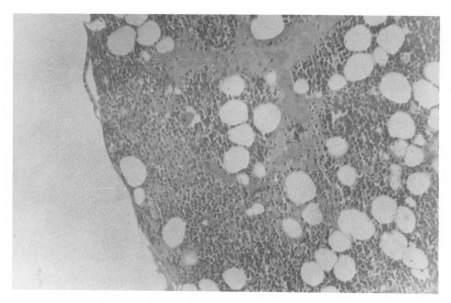

Fig. 5-9. Multiple myeloma (bone). Densely packed malignant plasma cells have invaded the marrow cavity (note fat cells), destroying normal bone tissue. (X100.)

cells that normally are found in lymphoid tissue and in bone marrow. The myeloma cells vary in size and shape and have a characteristic nucleus occupying an eccentric position in the cell. Normal plasma cells produce certain *gamma globulins* (antibodies), and myeloma cells may mimic this function. About 50% of patients with multiple myeloma have elevated levels of abnormal globulins in the blood and excrete Bence Jones protein (a low–molecular weight globulin) in the urine.

Histologically, the tumor shows closely packed malignant plasma cells infiltrating and eroding bone. The tumor is relatively radiosensitive to ionizing radiation (x-rays and gamma rays) and also responds well to some chemotherapeutic agents.

The leukemias

The characteristic feature of all leukemias is the uncontrolled and progressive overproduction of immature leukocytes (Figs. 5-10 to 5-12). In *myeloid* (myelogenous, granulocytic) leukemia, the predominant cells are granulocytic leukocytes. In lymphoid (lymphatic, lymphocytic) leukemia, the predominant cells are lymphocytes. In monocytic leukemia, the cells are monocytes. These classifications apply mainly to the chronic forms of the leukemias. The acute leukemias run a more rapid course and show a high percentage of very immature blood cells, or "blast" forms. In some acute leukemias, the malignant cells are so undifferentiated that it is impossible to distinguish between the myeloblastic (granulocytic) and lymphoblastic types. Acute leukemias are the most common cancers of children.

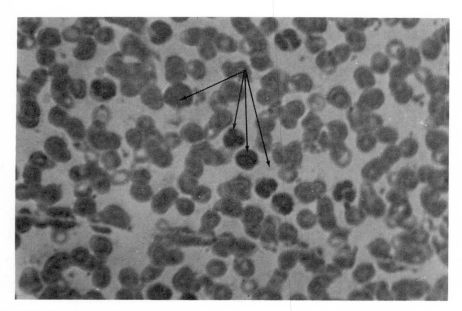

Fig. 5-10. Chronic granulocytic leukemia, peripheral blood. Abnormal increase in number of mature and immature neutrophils (*arrows*). (X400.)

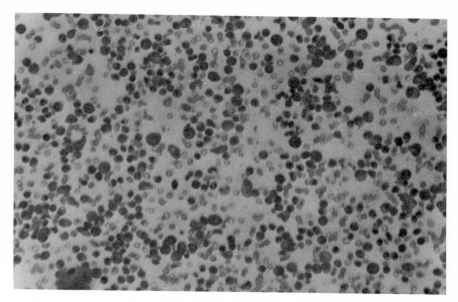

Fig. 5-11. Chronic granulocytic leukemia, bone marrow. Many myelocytes can be seen. (X100.)

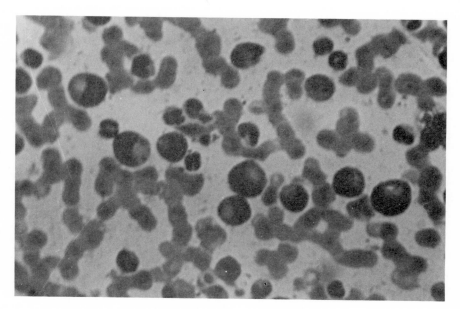

Fig. 5-12. Chronic granulocytic leukemia, bone marrow. (X400.) Cells are predominantly myelocytic. Normally, myelocytes constitute about 12% to 15% of bone marrow cells.

The bone marrow in all leukemias shows a massive replacement of the normal marrow cells by aggregates of proliferating leukemia cells. This replacement is responsible for the symptoms of anemia (lack of red blood cells) and thrombocytopenia (a lack of platelets leading to defective clotting of blood and a tendency to hemorrhage) that are commonly seen in patients with leukemia. In most cases, there is a marked increase in the number of circulating leukocytes of the type specific for the leukemia as well as many juvenile forms not normally seen in peripheral blood. Widespread infiltration of bone and other organs in the body usually occurs.

The leukemias have been the subject of much research. It has been shown that leukemias in fowls and mice are caused by viruses, but there is no proof that human leukemias are similarly caused. There is, however, some evidence that at least some of the human leukemias may be due to an acquired chromosomal defect. Chromosomes contain DNA, which programs the normal development of cells. In 1958, investigators found a tiny abnormal chromosome, the Philadelphia chromosome, replacing a normal chromosome in the leukocytes of patients with chronic myelogenous leukemia. The defective chromosome was apparently not inherited from either parent and was present only in the cells of the blood and bone marrow.

The causal relationship between exposure to total-body radiation and leukemia was dramatically demonstrated in the survivors of the atomic bomb explosions in Hiroshima and Nagasaki. In the decade following, these people showed a high incidence of the acute forms of leukemia, as well as chronic myelogenous leukemia. There was a direct relationship between the dose of atomic radiation received at the time of the explosion and the occurrence of the disease.

The treatment of people suffering from both the acute and the chronic leukemias has been significantly improved in recent years, due mainly to new radiotherapeutic techniques, the introduction of new chemotherapeutic drugs, and the use of the corticosteroid hormones.

6

Blood vessels and blood

Blood may be defined as a connective tissue with a fluid matrix. It is carried in a closed vascular (vessel) circuit and is pumped through the circuit by the heart. The system comprising the blood, blood vessels, and the heart is the circulatory system. Its primary function is transportation of various substances such as nutrients, wastes, respiratory gases, and hormones from one part of the body to another. In addition, the blood leukocytes play a vital role in the body's resistance to disease.

BLOOD VESSELS

The basic pattern of blood vessels shows a gradual progression from the smallest thinnest tubes, called *capillaries,* to vessels of increasing diameter and thicker walls. The larger vessels are either arteries or veins. The arteries are the distributing vessels leaving the heart and the veins are the collecting vessels returning blood to the heart.

The walls of all arteries and veins, large and small, are composed of three coats, or tunics: an internal lining *(tunica intima),* a middle layer *(tunica media),* and an outer covering *(tunica adventitia).* These tunics vary in structure and thickness in the different types of vessels. The most consistent feature of the tunica intima is the smooth glistening surface of endothelium lining the lumen of all vessels, as well as the heart. The tunica media is mainly smooth muscle, and the tunica adventitia is mainly loose fibroelastic connective tissue. The adventitia of large veins and arteries usually contains autonomic nerve endings, as well as *vasa vasorum* (vessels of the vessels), small networks of blood vessels supplying nutrients to the tissues of the wall.

The capillaries are the functioning portion of the circulatory system. A vast capillary network is found throughout the body tissues, and the exchange of substances between the blood and the tissues takes place across their walls. These tiny vessels form the link between the arterial and venous circulation. In general, they are about 8 to 10 microns in diameter. The wall is composed of a single layer of elongated endothelial cells (simple squamous epithelium) that show a conspicuous bulge at the center, where the nucleus is located. A thin basal lamina composed of collagen is usually present. Specialized capillaries, called sinusoids, are present in the liver, bone marrow, spleen, pituitary gland, and adrenal gland. These function as capillaries, but they have broad irregular lumina. They may be composed of true endothelium or, as in the liver, spleen, and bone marrow, the lining cells may consist of fixed macrophages of the reticuloendothelial system.

Arterial vessels have the thickest walls of the vascular system. The tunica intima is thickened by a subendothelial connective tissue layer containing elastic fibers, the internal elastic membrane. The tunica media is the thickest of the tunics, containing mainly smooth muscle in the smaller arteries and mainly elastic fibers in the larger arteries. The tunica adventitia may contain an external elastic membrane. Histologic sections of arterial vessels usually show a relatively thick wall and a small well-defined round lumen containing very little or no blood.

Veins have a larger and more irregular lumen than arteries, and are relatively thin-walled. Smooth muscle fibers are a constant feature in all the tunics; elastic fibers are usually found only in the larger veins. The tunica adventitia is the thickest part of the venous wall. Some veins contain valves, which appear as cusplike projections of the tunica intima into the lumen. In histologic sections, veins are often seen as partially collapsed vessels containing blood. The three tunics are not well defined, and the adventitia is usually the most prominent feature of the wall.

BLOOD

Blood is a fluid tissue that consists of a noncellular matrix called plasma and a cellular portion composed of *erythrocytes* (red blood cells) and *leukocytes* (white

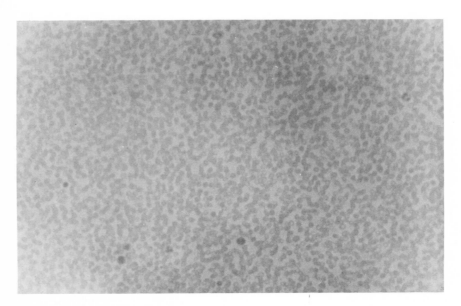

Fig. 6-1. Normal peripheral blood. (X100.) Compare the number of leukocytes seen in this field with Fig. 7-7.

blood cells). The total blood volume of an adult is about 5 liters, of which 55% is plasma and 45% is cells.

Plasma is a solution containing salts, plasma proteins, and varying amounts of other inorganic and organic substances. When blood vessel walls are damaged, the plasma protein, *fibrinogen,* is converted to a solid gel *(fibrin)*—the process of blood coagulation. The conversion of the fluid matrix to a solid prevents the excessive loss of blood from the body.

BLOOD CELLS (Figs. 6-1 and 6-2)
Erythrocytes

Human erythrocytes, or red blood cells, are nonnucleated biconcave disks about 8 microns in diameter. There are approximately 5,000,000 per cubic millimeter of blood, making a total of 25 million million (25 × 10^{12}) erythrocytes in an adult. The cells are small bags filled with a reddish iron-containing protein, *hemoglobin.* Hemoglobin transports most of the oxygen and about one third of the carbon dioxide used and produced by tissue metabolism. Erythrocytes are formed in the bone marrow and have a life span of about 120 days. Damaged and senile cells are removed from the blood stream by macrophages lining the sinusoids of the liver, spleen, and bone marrow.

Leukocytes

There are normally about 5,000 to 10,000 leukocytes per cubic millimeter of

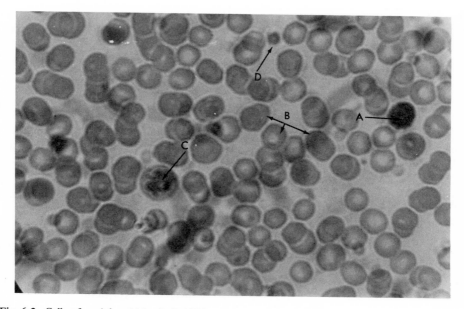

Fig. 6-2. Cells of peripheral blood. (×400.) *A*, Lymphocyte, *B*, red blood cells (erythrocytes), *C*, polymorphonuclear leukocyte, *D*, platelet.

blood. These are nucleated ameboid cells, which are classified as *granulocytes* (granular leukocytes) and *nongranulocytes* (nongranular leukocytes).

The granulocytes have two distinguishing features: the presence of abundant cytoplasmic granules, which give a specific staining reaction with polychrome blood stains such as Wright's stain, and the presence of a multilobed and complex nucleus. These cells are also called *polymorphonuclear leukocytes* (leukocytes containing nuclei of different shapes). There are three subgroups named on the basis of the staining reaction of the granules: *neutrophils* (containing fine inconspicuous granules, usually stained a lilac color), *eosinophils* (containing coarse red to orange granules), and *basophils* (containing very coarse dark blue granules). The nuclei of these cells are characteristically segmented and have three to five lobes connected by thin threads of chromatin. The number of lobes indicates the age of the cell. Juvenile forms, or band cells, have a horseshoe-shaped nucleus with no segmentation. Of the three groups, neutrophils are the most commonly found and make up about 65% of the leukocytes in adult peripheral blood. The cells are all actively mobile and phagocytic and function in the response of the body to invading microorganisms. The granules of basophils are known to contain the anticoagulant heparin and histamine. Granulocytes are formed in the bone marrow.

The nongranular leukocytes are the *lymphocytes,* which constitute about 25% of the leukocytes of adult peripheral blood, and the *monocytes*. The lymphocytes of peripheral blood are formed either in the bone marrow or in lymphoid tissue. Their structure and function are discussed in Chapter 7. Peripheral blood has about 5% monocytes, the largest white blood cells found in this tissue. The nucleus of these cells is usually indented and somewhat lighter staining than that of other leukocytes. The cytoplasm is abundant and stains a grayish blue. Monocytes are formed in the bone marrow. They are active phagocytes and are believed to be capable of diffentiating into tissue macrophages.

Also found in blood are small noncellular fragments called *platelets*. In stained blood smears, they appear as clumps of tiny oval or stellate blue disks. They are necessary for blood coagulation and hemostasis (limiting the escape of blood from damaged vessels). Platelets are formed by fragmentation of the cytoplasm of megakaryocytes in bone marrow.

ANEMIA

Anemia is a reduction in the number of circulating erythrocytes or the quantity of hemoglobin, or both. This condition may have many causes, among which are avitaminosis and malnutrition, iron deficiency, defects of the gastric mucosa *(pernicious anemia),* hemorrhage, diseases of the bone marrow, poisoning by toxic substances, autoimmune diseases, and hereditary defects. In anemic conditions, erythrocytes may show variations in size *(anisocytosis),* in shape *(poikilocytosis),* and in hemoglobin content *(hypochromia, hyperchromia).*

Sickle cell anemia (Fig. 6-3) is a hemolytic anemia caused by the inheritance of a

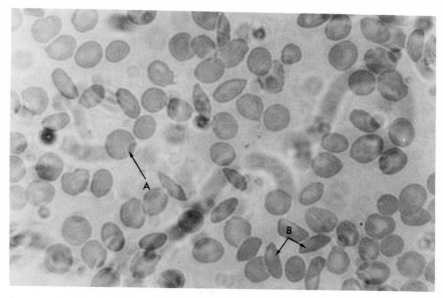

Fig. 6-3. Sickle cell anemia, peripheral blood. (X400.) Red blood cells show anisocytosis and poikilocytosis. *A*, Abnormally large erythrocytes (macrocytes), *B* sickle-shaped erythrocytes.

defective gene that controls the synthesis of hemoglobin. The defective hemoglobin produced in the body differs from normal hemoglobin in only a minor chemical detail, but this is sufficient to cause serious abnormalities in the red blood cells. In sickle cell anemia, erythrocytes tend to be larger and more fragile than their normal counterparts. When exposed to low oxygen tensions, the cells assume a characteristic sickle shape, which interferes with their passage through capillaries.

7

Lymphatic system

The lymphatic system consists of a fluid called lymph, the lymphatic vessels in which it flows, and various lymphoid tissues in the body, for example, lymph nodes and lymphoid organs such as the spleen and the thymus.

Lymph is composed mainly of interstitial fluid and solutes (including plasma proteins) that have diffused out of capillaries into the tissue spaces. The lymphatic vessels are, in effect, a one-way drainage system that collects this material and returns it to the blood. In addition to this vital function, lymphoid tissue is responsible for the production of antibodies and the body's resistance to disease.

LYMPHATIC VESSELS

The flow of lymph starts in branching networks of blind-ended lymphatic capillaries, which are widely distributed throughout the body. The walls of these capillaries are composed of a single layer of endothelium (simple squamous epithelium), as are those of the blood capillaries. However, they are larger and wider than blood capillaries, and the epithelium appears to lack a basement membrane. In the connective tissue core of the villi of the small intestine, large lymphatic capillaries, called *lacteals,* are specially adapted for the absorption of fat.

The lymphatic capillaries empty into larger lymphatic vessels, which resemble thin-walled veins in structure. As in veins, the walls consist of three coats, or tunics: an endothelial and elastic tissue tunica intima, and a tunica media and tunica adventitia, composed of varying amounts of smooth muscle and fibroelastic connective tissue. Unlike veins, the tunics of lymphatic vessels are not clearly outlined. Lymphatic vessels have numerous valves, formed by projections of the tunica intima. A characteristic feature of lymphatic vessels is that they drain through lymph nodes at intervals along their route.

The largest lymphatic trunks are the *thoracic* and *right lymphatic ducts,* which empty the lymph drained from all areas of the body into the brachiocephalic (innominate) veins at the base of the neck. The walls of these ducts are thicker than those of other lymphatic vessels and contain an internal elastic membrane and bundles of longitudinal and circular smooth muscle in the tunica media.

LYMPHOID TISSUE

Lymphoid tissue is diffusely distributed in the lamina propria of mucous membranes, mainly of the alimentary, respiratory, and urinary tracts. In the *ileum,* well-defined aggregates of lymphoid tissue called Peyer's patches can be seen in the lamina propria (Fig. 7-1). In the pharynx there are three major lymphoid aggregates, or tonsils; these, in addition to such distinct structures as the lymph nodes, spleen, and thymus, can be considered lymphoid organs.

Lymphocytes

The cell common to all lymphoid tissue is the *lymphocyte.* The typical lymphocyte has a large, round or slightly indented nucleus with dark, clumped chromatin and variable amounts of pale blue basophilic cytoplasm. The cells may be small, medium, or large. The small lymphocytes appear to be composed almost entirely of nucleus; very little cytoplasm can be seen. The larger lymphocytes have a paler staining nucleus and more abundant cytoplasm. In lymphoid tissue, the larger lymphocytes are located in a pale-staining *germinal center,* which is surrounded by a dark-staining zone of small lymphocytes. Larger lymphocytes usually remain in lymphoid tissue; small lymphocytes circulate from lymphatic structures into lymph and into the blood stream, where they comprise about 30% of the total leukocyte count. They are also capable of leaving the blood and moving into tissue spaces. Large numbers of these lymphocytes are often seen at sites of inflammation and infection in the body.

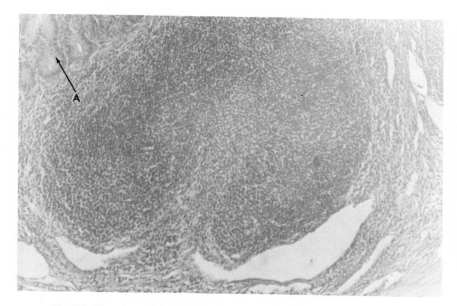

Fig. 7-1. Peyer's patch in intestinal mucosa. (X100.) *A,* Mucosal epithelium.

The origin of lymphocytes is not entirely clear, but it is probable that lymphoid stem cells in the bone marrow produce the 10% to 20% of lymphocytes normally found in marrow. These stem cells also emigrate to the thymus, where they differentiate into thymic lymphocytes. Marrow lymphocytes and thymic lymphocytes in turn populate the other lymphoid tissues of the body and are able to undergo mitosis and increase their numbers in these tissues. A few lymphocytes have a short life span of about a week; the majority apparently live for years.

Certain lymphocytes can differentiate to form plasma cells. These are deeply basophilic cells with a small eccentric (off center) nucleus. The function of lymphocytes and plasma cells is to produce antibodies.

LYMPHOID ORGANS
Lymph nodes

Chains of lymph nodes are found in various regions of the body, such as the axilla, neck, mesentery, mediastinum, and the inguinal region (groin). These small bean-shaped structures are adapted for the filtration of lymph, *lymphopoiesis* (production of lymphocytes), and the production of antibodies. Afferent lymphatic vessels enter each node at its wider convex surface; efferent lymphatic vessels drain the node at the hilus, an indentation on the opposite surface. Lymph nodes are enclosed in a capsule of dense collagenous connective tissue, which extends inward in strands, or trabeculae. The fibrous trabeculae intermingle with a fine meshwork of reticular fibers, making up the stroma (supporting framework) of the node.

The reticular fibers are part of the reticular connective tissue component of lymphoid tissue. The reticular cells of this connective tissue are stellate-shaped basophilic cells with large pale nuclei. Reticular cells can develop into fixed and free tissue macrophages, which are ameboid and phagocytic.

The interior of the node is divided into an outer *cortex* and an inner *medulla*, located mainly around the hilus. The cortical area consists of rounded *follicles,* or *nodules* (small nodes), and numerous *sinuses,* or spaces, through which the lymph filters. The follicles are aggregates of lymphoid tissue separated from each other by connective tissue trabeculae (Fig. 7-2). Some may show a dark-staining peripheral zone of packed small lymphocytes and a more lightly stained *germinal center* composed of medium and large lymphocytes. The nodules are not permanent structures and tend to grow or regress depending on the needs of the organism. In the medulla, which is not sharply demarcated from the cortex, the lymphoid tissue is arranged in cords surrounded by sinuses. The lymph sinuses are irregular channels lined by reticular cells and macrophages. A constant flow of lymph, emptying from the afferent lymphatic vessels, trickles through the subcapsular sinuses into the cortical and medullary sinuses and is then collected by the efferent lymphatics at the hilus. As it passes through the spaces of the node, the lymph is cleared of particles such as dust, carbon, bacteria, and cellular debris by the phagocytic reticular cells. In addition, antibody is produced when necessary, and small lymphocytes of the node enter the lymph stream.

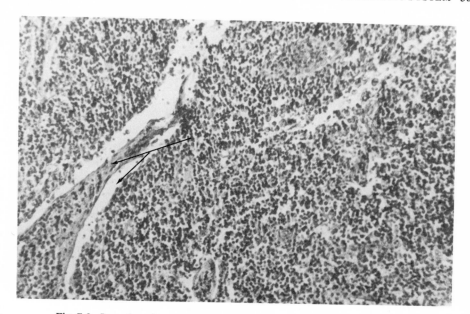

Fig. 7-2. Lymph node, cortex. Trabecula and cortical sinus (*arrows*). (×100.)

Tonsils

The tonsils are well-defined collections of lymphoid tissue situated beneath the surface epithelium of the pharynx. Three groups of tonsils form a protective ring at the opening to the respiratory and digestive tracts; these are the paired *palatine tonsils* lying on each side of the entrance to the throat, the *lingual tonsil* at the root of the tongue, and the *pharyngeal tonsil* (adenoids) on the dorsal wall of the nasopharynx. The structure of the three tonsillar masses is similar except that stratified squamous epithelium overlies the palatine and lingual tonsils, wheras the surface epithelium over the pharyngeal tonsil is mainly ciliated pseudostratified columnar. The epithelium is a continuation of the mucosal epithelium of the oropharynx and the nasopharynx, respectively.

The lymphoid tissue of the tonsillar masses in the lamina propria is arranged in nodules with or without germinal centers. A loose capsule of fibrous connective tissue covers the base of the lymphoid tissue and forms irregular septa (partitions) between the nodules.

Histologic features of the tonsils are the presence of crypts (pockets), lined by the surface epithelium, which extend deep into the lymphoid tissue, and the presence of mucous or mixed seromucous glands in the pharyngeal submucosa below the capsule.

Thymus

The thymus is a flat bilobed gland located in the anterior mediastinum above the heart. The two longitudinal lobes are joined together by fibrous connective tissue. This tissue also forms the capsule surrounding the lobes and extends septa into the gland, dividing the lobes into thousands of lobules.

Each lobule is further subdivided into a peripheral dark-staining cortex around a light-staining medulla. The medullary tissue of the lobules is continuous, with a core of light-staining tissue in the center of the gland.

The parenchyma of an active thymus is composed mainly of two cell types, lymphocytes (small, medium, and large) and odd-branching stellate cells of epithelial origin. The latter resemble reticular cells in appearance, but the characteristic reticular fibers are absent. These epithelioreticular elements interconnect with each other by means of cytoplasmic processes, thus forming an extensive network, or cytoreticulum (a network composed of cells rather than fibers), the spaces of which are filled with lymphocytes. The cortex is so densely packed with lymphocytes that the epithelioreticular network is not easily seen (Fig. 7-3). In the medullary areas, however, lymphocytes are less numerous, and the large eosinophilic epithelioreticular cells with pale nuclei are more evident. The central medullary area also contains *thymic corpuscles* (Hassall's corpuscles), which are a characteristic feature of the thymus. These are round nests of flattened acidophilic epithelial cells arranged in concentric layers. The cells at the center of Hassall's corpuscles often undergo degeneration, with the formation of small cystic spaces.

The thymus lacks afferent lymphatics and lymph sinuses, but is supplied with blood vessels and efferent lymphatic vessels.

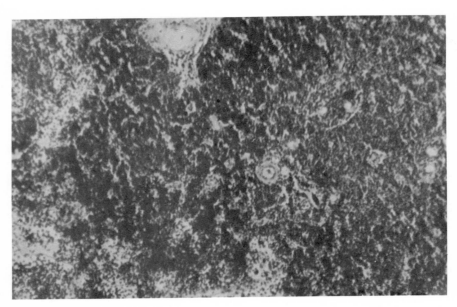

Fig. 7-3. Thymus; dense aggregates of small lymphocytes in cortex. (X100.)

The gland is most active in young animals. It is believed that thymic lymphocytes populate the lymph nodes and the spleen and are responsible for the development and the immunologic competence of lymphoid tissue throughout the body. In addition, the thymus appears to secrete a hormonal substance that stimulates the production of lymphocytes.

Spleen

The spleen is the largest lymphoid organ in the body (Fig. 7-4). It is located in the upper left portion of the abdomen, between the stomach and the diaphragm. It is covered by a thin capsule of fibroelastic connective tissue containing some smooth muscle cells. The capsule is in turn covered by a layer of peritoneal mesothelium. The connective tissue is thickest at the hilus, a deep medial indentation where blood vessels, lymphatics, and nerves enter and leave the spleen. The stroma (supporting framework) of the spleen consists of thick branching trabeculae, which dip down from the capsule and contain numerous elastic fibers. The larger trabeculae are visible to the naked eye. The fibers of the trabeculae are continous with a diffuse network of reticular connective tissue within the organ. The spleen is a highly vascular organ with an extensive arterial and venous supply.

The parenchyma consists of areas of white pulp and red pulp. The *white pulp* is formed by lymphocytes of various sizes, which fill the spaces in the mesh of reticular fibers. Associated with the lymphocytes are plasma cells, reticular cells, and

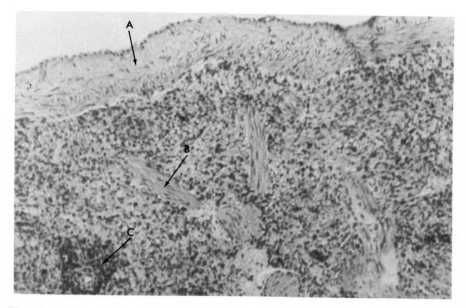

Fig. 7-4. Spleen. *A*, Splenic capsule, *B*, trabecula, *C*, splenic nodule with central artery. (X100.)

macrophages. The white pulp forms cylindrical strands around some of the splenic arterioles, as well as aggregates of nodular lymphoid tissue, the splenic nodules. These nodules contain an eccentrically placed central artery and a germinal center. The *red pulp* forms a diffuse mass around the splenic nodules and is a modified form of the lymphoid tissue of the white pulp. It is traversed by a system of venous sinuses lined by endothelium. Cords of cells lie between the sinuses. The splenic cords contain connective tissue cells, red and white blood cells, and macrophages.

The spleen has several functions. It serves as a reservoir for red blood cells, which are retained in the red pulp. These cells can apparently be released into the circulation by contraction of the smooth muscle elements in the capsule and the trabeculae. The spleen produces lymphocytes, plasma cells, and antibodies; in fetal life, it acts as a hemopoietic organ. The macrophages of the spleen actively filter blood passing through the sinuses, removing senile and damaged erythrocytes and platelets, particulate material, and bacteria.

INVOLUTION OF LYMPHOID TISSUE

Most lymphoid tissue in man undergoes a decrease in size and activity after puberty. This process of involution is particularly marked in the thymus, which becomes atrophic (shrunken) and infiltrated by fat cells. The tonsils also tend to atrophy and become fibrotic (infiltrated by fibrous connective tissue) after puberty. In the adult, many lymph nodes lack germinal centers and have reduced numbers of lymphocytes. However, this picture is variable, and nodes may regenerate and become active in the presence of infection.

The lymphocytic cells of lymphoid tissues and organs are very sensitive to adrenal glucocorticoid hormones and ionizing radiation such as x-rays. The administration of cortisol (or ACTH from the adenohypophysis, which stimulates the secretion of cortisol from the adrenal cortex) destroys large numbers of lymphocytes and causes involution of lymphoid structures. X-radiation has a similar, rapidly destructive effect on lymphocytes and lymphoid tissue, as do certain radiomimetic chemicals such as the nitrogen mustards.

TUMORS OF LYMPHOID ORIGIN
Hodgkin's disease

Hodgkin's disease, complex in nature, has the characteristics of a malignant process in lymph nodes. It is believed by some to be caused by a virus, although the evidence for this is doubtful. Hodgkin's disease occurs most often in men in the age group 30 to 50, and less frequently occurs in children. The affected lymph nodes may show a wide range of histologic changes (Fig. 7-5). These include proliferation of atypical lymphocytes and reticular cells, inflammatory reactions characterized by the presence of fibroblasts, plasma cells, and polymorphonuclear leukocytes (particularly eosinophils), *necrosis* (death of normal tissue in the nodes), and *fibrosis* (replacement of normal tissue in the nodes by fibrous tissue). The diagnosis of Hodgkin's disease

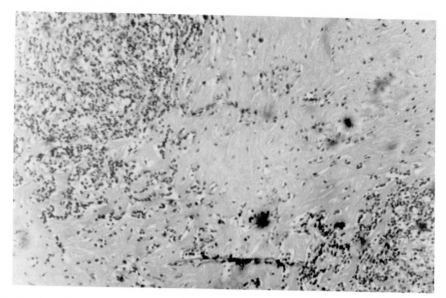

Fig. 7-5. Lymph node in Hodgkin's disease. Bands of fibrous connective tissue separate islands of proliferating lymphoid cells. (X100.)

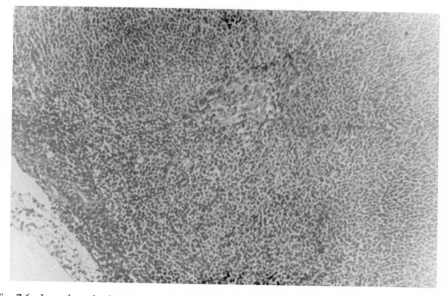

Fig. 7-6. Lymph node; lymphosarcoma. Node is overrun by masses of small lymphocytes. (X100.)

depends on the presence of *Sternberg-Reed cells,* giant cells with multilobed nuclei and prominent nucleoli. These bizarre cells probably arise from reticular cells. The progress of the disease is variable. In certain cases it may remain confined to the lymph nodes for long periods; in others, there may be widespread infiltration of the bone marrow, bones, skin, and viscera.

Hodgkin's disease is radiosensitive, and even advanced cases show a favorable response to treatment with adequate doses of x-rays.

Lymphosarcoma

Lymphosarcoma is a tumor of lymphoid tissue, composed of malignant cells similar to small lymphocytes (Fig. 7-6). The tumor most commonly arises in lymph nodes, tonsils, and lymphoid tissue of the gastrointestinal tract. Histologically, the lymphoid tissue is overrun by malignant small lymphocytes, and its normal architecture is destroyed. The invasion of lymphatics and veins can lead to metastases in the liver, lung, and skeleton.

Like lymphoid tissue generally, lymphosarcoma is radiosensitive, and the treatment of choice in this condition is radiation therapy.

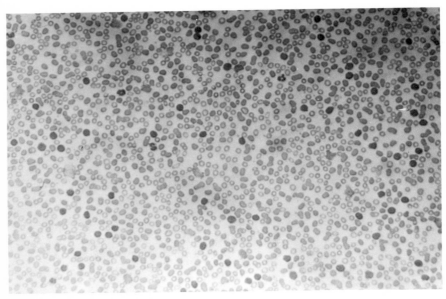

Fig. 7-7. Lymphocytic leukemia, peripheral blood. The lymphocytes have dark-staining nuclei with little or no cytoplasm. Only a few neutrophils are present. This low-power field would normally show no more than five leukocytes, mainly neutrophils. The red blood cells show hypochromia and anisocytosis, indicating anemia. (X100.)

Chronic lymphocytic (lymphatic) leukemia

Chronic lymphocytic leukemia is a malignant disease characterized by the uncontrolled proliferation of abnormal lymphocytes in lymphoid organs, bone marrow, and circulating blood. Smears of bone marrow and peripheral blood show abnormally large numbers of lymphocytes (Fig. 7-7). These cells replace the normal components of bone marrow (causing anemia and hemorrhage due to insufficient platelets) and infiltrate the gastrointestinal tract, brain, liver, and kidneys.

This leukemia responds well to x-radiation, various antitumor drugs, and the adrenal corticoid hormones.

For additional discussion of the leukemias, see Chapter 5.

8

Digestive system

The digestive system is essentially a tube about 30 feet long, extending from the mouth to the anus. The parts of the digestive tract are the mouth, pharynx, esophagus, stomach, small intestine, and large intestine. Three accessory glands of digestion, the major salivary glands, the liver, and the pancreas, are found outside the tube, but empty their digestive juices through ducts into the tract.

MOUTH

The interior of the oral cavity is lines by moist stratified squamous epithelium. In some areas, such as the gums (gingivae) and the hard palate, the stratified squamous epithelium is keratinized and closely resembles the epidermis. In the cheeks, soft palate, and floor of the mouth the epithelium is nonkeratinized. The lamina propria varies from fibroelastic to reticular connective tissue and is thrown up into characteristic ridges or papillae. A submucosa composed of connective tissue and fat cells is present in the cheeks and the soft palate. Many mucous and mixed seromucous glands, which keep the oral cavity moist, are found deep in the connective tissue layers. In the movable portions of the mouth there is a muscularis layer composed of skeletal muscle. In other regions the connective tissue lamina is attached directly to bone.

The human adult has 32 permanent teeth, each of which is composed of a visible portion, the crown, and an embedded portion, the root. The roots lie in bony sockets, or *alveoli,* of the upper and lower jaw *(maxilla* and *mandible).* The crown is covered by a very hard, noncellular, calcified material called *enamel.* The center of each tooth, the *pulp cavity,* is filled with specialized connective tissue containing small blood vessels and nerves. The pulp cavity is enclosed in *dentin,* a hard tissue resembling bone.

The tongue is a mobile and muscular organ composed of bundles of interlacing skeletal muscle covered by thick keratinized stratified squamous epithelium on the upper surface and nonkeratinized epithelium on the under surface. The epithelium rests on a dense fibrous connective tissue lamina propria, which extends downward into the muscle bundles. The lamina propria of the upper surface of the tongue is thrown up into very tall papillae that are visible to the naked eye. Many mucous, serous, and mixed glands can be seen in the lamina. Embedded in the epithelium are taste buds, small oval clusters of pale-staining neuroepithelial cells. The taste buds communicate with nerve fibers at their base. An aggregate of lymphoid tissue, the lingual tonsil, is present below the epithelium at the root of the tongue.

PHARYNX

The pharynx, or throat, is a pathway for both food and air. It is subdivided into three parts: the nasopharynx, which communicates with the nasal passages and is a part of the respiratory tract; the oropharynx, which extends from the soft palate of the roof of the mouth to the hyoid bone; and the laryngopharynx, between the hyoid bone and the esophagus.

The oropharynx and laryngopharynx, contain an inner mucosa composed of stratified squamous epithelium and a fibroelastic connective tissue lamina propria. In the lamina are found small mucous glands, as well as aggregates of lymphoid tissue, which in the oropharynx are called the palatine tonsils. Below the lamina is a muscular coat, or tunic, consisting of two layers of skeletal muscle.

DESIGN OF THE DIGESTIVE TUBE

The digestive tract, from the esophagus to the anus, is a hollow tube, the wall of which is composed of four concentric layers or tunics of tissue. These are, in sequence from the innermost (luminal) surface to the outer surface, the (tunica) *mucosa,* the (tunica or tela) *submucosa,* the (tunica) *muscularis,* and the (tunica) *adventitia,* or *serosa.*

The mucosa, or mucous membrane, consists of three distinct zones: a surface epithelium, a *lamina propria* below the epithelium, composed of areolar or reticular connective tissue (or a mixture of both), and a thin *muscularis mucosae* composed usually of an inner circular and an outer longitudinal arrangement of smooth muscle fibers. The lamina propria of the digestive tract may contain various glands, as well as accumulations of lymphoid tissue.

The submucosa, which is situated below the muscularis mucosae, is a coarse fibroelastic connective tissue layer containing large blood vessels, lymphatics, and nerves. It may also contain large aggregates of lymphoid tissue and deep glands that extend downward from the mucosa.

Below the submucosa, the muscularis consists mainly of two relatively thick layers of muscle, the inner layer being circular and the outer layer longitudinal. Neurons of autonomic ganglia lie between the two layers. For the most part, the muscle is smooth muscle, except for the upper quarter of the esophagus and the external anal sphincter, where it is striated.

The outermost coat, or adventitia, is generally fibrous connective tissue. In those parts of the digestive tract that are within the abdominal cavity, the outermost coat is formed by folds of the peritoneum and is called a serosa. The serosa is composed of mesothelium (simple squamous epithelium) lying on a delicate lamina propria of areolar connective tissue.

The structure of the four tunics is modified in various ways at different levels of the alimentary tube. In the following sections, only special aspects that are characteristic of each region of the digestive tract will be discussed.

ESOPHAGUS

The esophagus is a tube about 10 inches long, which connects the pharynx to the stomach. It runs from the neck, through the mediastinum of the thoracic cavity (behind the trachea), and ends just below the diaphragm.

The mucosal epithelium consists of a thick layer of highly stratified nonkeratinized squamous cells. The muscularis mucosae is composed only of longitudinally arranged fibers and is the thickest in the entire digestive tube. Mucosal and submucosal mucus-secreting glands occur, but are not very numerous. The tunica muscularis contains skeletal muscle in the upper portion of the esophagus, mixed skeletal and smooth muscle in the middle portion, and smooth muscle in the lower portion. At the junction of the esophagus and the stomach, the smooth muscle forms a circular band, the cardiac sphincter. The external tunic of the esophagus throughout most of its length is a loose fibrous connective tissue adventitia. The short segment of the esophagus below the diaphragm is covered with serosa.

STOMACH

The stomach is a dilated part of the digestive tube, extending from the left side of the upper abdominal cavity, where it is continuous with the esophagus, to the right

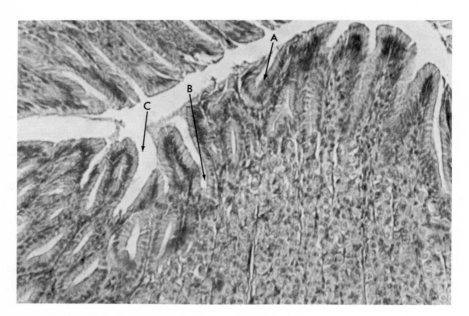

Fig. 8-1 Stomach. *A*, Gastric epithelium, *B*, gastric gland, *C*, gastric pits. (×100.)

side where it is continuous with the duodenum of the small intestine. The area around the *cardiac sphincter* is called the *cardia,* and the narrowed area around the opening *(pylorus)* to the duodenum is called the *pyloric region.* The rest of the stomach is called the *body,* or corpus. That portion of the body that bulges above the cardiac orifice is called the *fundus.* The mucosa and submucosa of the stomach are thrown up into deep folds, or *rugae,* which disappear when the stomach is distended.

The surface of the entire gastric mucosa is simple tall columnar epithelium (Fig. 8-1). This lining dips down to form many narrow deep furrows, or *gastric pits,* also known as *foveolae.* Branched tubular glands empty into the base of each pit. In the pyloric region, the pits are deeper than in the cardia and body. The pyloric and cardiac glands are coiled and mainly mucus secreting. The glands in the body and fundus of the stomach, which are called fundic or gastric glands, are straight tubular glands containing three distinct cell types. In the neck of the glands are found pale-staining *mucous neck cells* that secrete mucus. Between the mucous neck cells are large

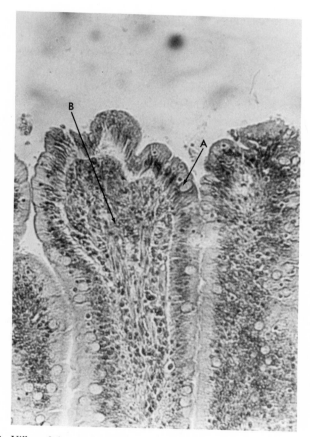

Fig. 8-2. Villus of the small intestine. *A,* Goblet cell, *B,* lamina propria. (X100.)

acidophilic *parietal cells* that secrete hydrochloric acid. The cells at the lower portions of the glands are pyramid-shaped granular cells called *chief cells*. The granules of the chief cells are composed of pepsinogen, a precursor of the gastric juice enzyme, pepsin.

The muscularis of the stomach consists of three thick layers of smooth muscle, an inner oblique layer, a middle circular layer, and an outer longitudinal layer. At the junction of the stomach and the duodenum, the circular muscle is thickened and forms the pyloric sphincter, which controls the amount of gastric contents that are emptied into the small intestine.

SMALL INTESTINE

The small intestine is an extensively coiled tube about 20 feet long. It is divided into a short upper portion, the *duodenum,* which is about 10 inches long, a central *jejunum* about 8 feet long, and a terminal portion, the *ileum,* about 12 feet in length.

Since the absorption of food materials takes place in the small intestine, the surface area for absorption is greatly increased in several ways: (1) the mucosa and submucosa of the small intestine are thrown up into permanent circular folds called the *plicae circulares;* (2) the mucosa of the small intestine is arranged in numerous fingerlike elevations, or *villi,* which make the surface velvety; and (3) the simple tall columnar epithelial cells lining the small intestine have many tiny projecting *microvilli* on the surface facing the lumen. These microvilli are so numerous that they appear as a brush border.

The villi vary somewhat in height and shape in different segments of the small intestine (Fig. 8-2). Each villus consists of a central core of the connective tissue lamina propria, covered by a single layer of columnar epithelium containing many goblet cells. Within each villus is an arteriole, a capillary network, a venule, and a lymphatic vessel called a *lacteal*.

Between the villi are many simple tubular glands that extend from the muscularis mucosae to the surface. These are known as the intestinal glands, or *crypts of Lieberkühn,* and are made up of mucus-secreting simple tall columnar cells. At the base of the crypts are pyramidal Paneth cells with acidophilic granules in the cytoplasm. Paneth cells probably secrete digestive enzymes.

The submucosa of the duodenum differs from the rest of the small intestine in that it contains clusters of compound tubular mucus-secreting glands known as *Brunner's glands*. These glands are absent elsewhere in the small intestine.

Patches of lymphoid tissue are commonly found in the mucosa of the small and large intestines. Aggregate lymph nodules, Peyer's patches, are found mainly in the ileum and the appendix (see Fig. 7-1). These nodules are part of the immune system of the body.

LARGE INTESTINE

The large intestine is a tube about 5 feet long. It extends from the *ileocecal valve,* a smooth muscle sphincter at the junction of the ileum and the cecum, to the anus. It consists of a blind pouch called the *cecum;* an ascending, transverse, and descending colon; a *sigmoid* (S-shaped) section of the colon; the rectum, or terminal portion of the colon; and the anus, or external opening of the colon.

The surface epithelium of the large intestine is identical to that of the small intestine and contains many goblet cells. There are, however, no villi and no plicae circulares. The crypts of Lieberkühn, consisting mainly of tall mucus-secreting cells, are longer and more closely packed than those of the small intestine. The lamina propria contains many single lymphatic nodules that can extend into the submucosa. The appendix, which is a wormlike projection of the cecum, is characterized by large amounts of lymphoid tissue in the wall and, in fact, resembles a lymphoid organ.

The longitudinal muscle fibers of the muscularis layer of most of the large intestine are gathered into thick bands called the *taeniae coli.* The taeniae are shorter than the intestinal wall and cause it to bulge. These bulges form the characteristic *haustra* of the large intestine. Between the haustra, semilunar folds, or *plicae semilunares,* can be seen on the inside surface of the colon.

The rectum at the end of the colon lacks the taeniae. At the terminal portion of the rectum, and the anal canal with which it is continuous, the serosa is replaced by an adventitia.

The anal canal differs from the rest of the large intestine. The epithelium changes from simple columnar to stratified cuboidal, and finally to stratified squamous containing hair follicles, sweat glands, and sebaceous glands as it merges with the epidermis at the anal orifice. The muscularis mucosae disappears. The submucosa of the anal canal contains a large plexus of hemorrhoidal veins. The circular layer of the muscularis thickens to form the involuntary internal anal sphincter. At the anal orifice, skeletal muscle fibers form the external anal sphincter.

TUMORS OF THE GASTROINTESTINAL TRACT
Adenocarcinoma of the stomach

The mucosal lining of the stomach dips down to form long tubular glands composed of simple columnar cells that secrete mucus and cells that secrete the other components of gastric juice. The most common neoplasm of the stomach arises from this epithelium and is classified as an adenocarcinoma (Fig. 8-3). The tumor cells may be well differentiated or anaplastic (a loss of normal appearance and function). The most common site of occurrence is the prepyloric region of the stomach. The neoplastic cells form glandular structures that are irregular and disorganized. The normal position of the nuclei at the base of each columnar cell is changed, and the malignant cells appear pseudostratified. The edges of the tumor are thickened, and the central portion often ulcerates. There is a rapid invasion of the thickness of the stomach wall from the mucosa to the serosa and a spread to neighboring structures such as the omentum and the pancreas. The tumor characteristically spreads to regional lymph nodes and from these to distant organs by way of the lymphatics.

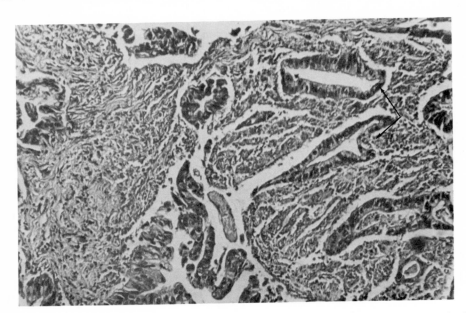

Fig. 8-3. Fairly well-differentiated adenocarcinoma of the stomach, showing malignant glands (*arrows*) invading stomach wall. (×100.)

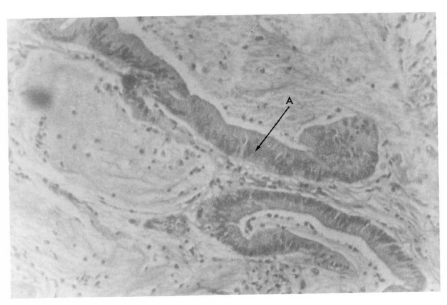

Fig. 8-4. Adenocarcinoma of the large intestine. *A*, Tall dark-staining malignant columnar cells appear pseudostratified. (×100.)

Although the cause of the tumor is unknown, there is some evidence that chronic gastric ulcers, pernicious anemia, and genetic factors may predispose to it.

Adenocarcinoma of the intestine

Cancer of the intestinal mucosa can occur anywhere along the entire tract, but most frequently involves the sigmoid colon and the rectum; 80% of all intestinal tumors occur in this region. The cecum, ascending colon, and ileum are affected less frequently, and the jejunum and duodenum rarely are. The tumor cells are derived from the simple columnar epithelium of the crypts of Lieberkühn. The neoplastic cells are taller and stain more intensely than to the normal columnar mucosal cells (Fig. 8-4). The nuclei no longer occupy the base of the cells, thus giving the appearance of pseudostratification. The malignant crypts are irregularly shaped and can be seen invading the lamina propria, muscularis mucosae, and submucosa. The circular and longitudinal smooth muscle layers and the lymphatic network between them are often infiltrated by tumor cells. These tumors spread by way of the lymphatics to distant lymph nodes and through the veins to the liver, lungs, kidneys, and the brain.

ACCESSORY DIGESTIVE GLANDS
Major salivary glands

There are three paired salivary glands that empty their secretion, saliva, into the mouth. These are the *parotid glands* (Fig. 8-5), which lie in front of the external ear;

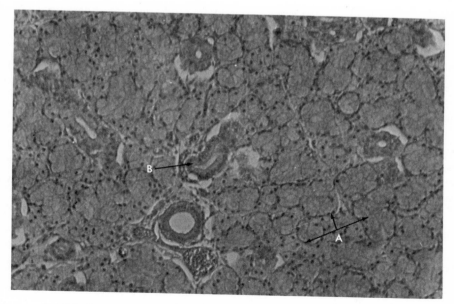

Fig. 8-5. Parotid gland. *A*, Serous alveoli, *B*, excretory duct (striated). (X100.)

the *submandibular glands* in the floor of the mouth; and the *sublingual glands,* which lie near the central mucosal fold in the floor of the mouth.

The salivary glands are compound *tubuloacinar glands* enclosed in fibrous connective tissue capsules that extend inward to form septa, dividing the glands into lobes and smaller lobules. Within the lobules, the branching glandular structures are embedded in a fine reticular connective tissue stroma. The glandular elements are secretory cells arranged in acini and tubules. A series of ducts of increasing size, ranging from intercalated ducts to larger secretory ducts to excretory ducts, drains the secretions of the glandular cells. The main excretory duct of each salivary gland opens into the mouth.

Acini composed of serous cells, mucous cells, and a mixture of both are characteristic of the salivary glands. The purely serous acini secrete a clear, rather watery fluid containing the enzyme *salivary amylase* (ptyalin), which is involved in the digestion of starch. These acini are composed of a single layer of pyramidal cells with dark-staining granular cytoplasm. The nuclei are oval and are located at the base of the cell. The purely mucous acini secrete a thick mucoid substance that contains no enzyme. The cells are arranged in a single layer and are wedge-shaped, with flattened nuclei at the base. The cytoplasm is usually filled with mucigen, but after histologic processing this material may be dissolved out. The cells thus appear to be spongy or honeycombed, with many empty spaces. In the mixed acini, the serous cells form crescent-shaped caps (demilunes) at the rounded end of the acinus, whereas the mucous cells are arranged at the neck, closest to the opening of the intercalated duct. The serous cells of a demilune are smaller in size than the mucous cells.

In man, the parotid gland is purely serous (Fig. 8-5), and the submandibular and sublingual glands are mixed seromucous.

Scattered *basket cells,* or *myoepithelial cells,* are commonly found in the secretory endpieces and in the small intercalated ducts leading from them. These are thin, flat cells with numerous cytoplasmic processes, which encircle the secreting elements. They are believed to be capable of contraction, and thus propel the secretions into the ducts.

The smallest of the intralobular ducts, the intercalated ducts, are composed of simple low cuboidal epithelium. The secretory ducts, next in size, are lined by tall acidophilic columnar epithelium, with well-defined vertical striations at the base of the cells. These ducts, also called *striated ducts,* are a characteristic feature of the salivary glands, particularly the parotid and the submandibular.

Excretory ducts of varying sizes are found outside of the lobules. They are lined with simple columnar epithelium that gradually changes to pseudostratified columnar and then to stratified columnar epithelium. Near the main outlet of the gland, the walls of the excretory ducts are composed of stratified squamous epithelium.

The liver

The liver (Fig. 8-6) is the largest gland in the body. It occupies the upper right quadrant of the abdominal cavity, just below the diaphragm. It is made up of

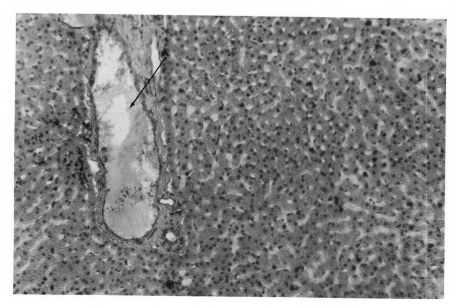

Fig. 8-6. Liver. *A*, Hepatic lobule with bile duct. (✗100.)

four lobes that are partially connected and hundreds of small polygonal *lobules,* which are the structural units of the organ. The lobules are separated from each other by thin strands of connective tissue.

Hepatic lobule. The center of each lobule is occupied by a small vein called the *central vein.* Hepatic cells, arranged in *cords,* extend radially, like the spokes of a wheel, from the central vein outward to the periphery of the lobule. The highly specialized glandular epithelium of the liver consists of large many-sided cells, with a single large nucleus, although binucleate and multinucleate cells may also be present. The cytoplasm is granular and contains variable amounts of glycogen granules, fat droplets, protein granules, and bile pigments. Two types of vessels are intimately associated with the cords of hepatic cells. The first of these are the *bile canaliculi,* extremely small tubules that collect bile from the cells and carry it to the interlobular *bile ducts* at the periphery of the lobules. The second are the *hepatic sinusoids,* specialized very thin-walled capillary-type blood vessels that have wide and irregularly shaped lumina. Blood in the hepatic sinusoids flows into the central vein. Sinusoids are lined with thin endothelium interspersed with odd stellate-shaped, actively phagocytic cells—*Kupffer cells.* These macrophages are part of the reticuloendothelial system of the body, which is concerned with resistance to disease and the removal of cellular debris. The arrangement of this duct and blood vessel system provides two outlets for the secretions of the liver cells; the canaliculi collect the bile secreted by the cells and the sinusoids enable the liver cells to secrete glucose, plasma proteins, and other essential substances directly into the blood stream.

At the edges of the lobules, where two or three lobules meet, there is a larger area of well-defined interlobular connective tissue called the *portal area*. Embedded in each portal area is a characteristic thin-walled branch of the hepatic portal vein, a small thick-walled branch of the hepatic artery, and one or more bile ducts lined with cuboidal to low columnar epithelium with a thin connective tissue base.

Gallbladder

The gallbladder is a small pear-shaped organ with a single duct, the cystic duct, leading from it, which joins the main hepatic duct, coming from the liver, to form the common bile duct. The gallbladder functions as a reservoir for bile.

The wall consists of several layers (Fig. 8-7). The mucosa is composed of simple tall columnar epithelial cells, with a lamina propria of vascular connective tissue. There are no goblet cells or glands. The mucosa is thrown up into deep folds, which tend to disappear when the gallbladder is distended. The muscular coat is a thin irregular

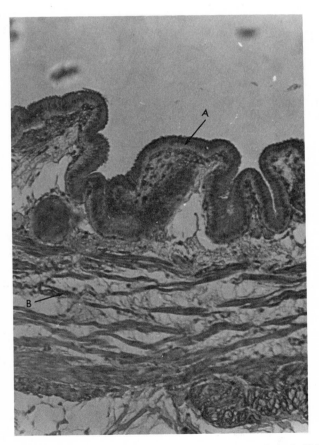

Fig. 8-7. Gallbladder . *A*, Columnar epithelium, *B*, muscularis. (X100.)

network of circular smooth muscle fibers and some collagenous, reticular, and elastic fibers. Below the muscularis is a thick, loose connective tissue layer, covered by an adventitia on the portions of the gallbladder that are near the liver, and a serosa elsewhere.

Extrahepatic ducts

There are three large bile ducts outside the liver. These are the *hepatic duct* from the liver, the *cystic duct* from the gallbladder, and the *common bile duct* formed by the union of the first two ducts. The common bile duct empties into the duodenum, usually jointly with the pancreatic duct. The ducts are lined with simple tall columnar epithelium and have a fibroelastic connective tissue wall with occasional areas of smooth muscle. At the junction of the common duct, the pancreatic duct, and the duodenum, a circular ring of smooth muscle forms Oddi's sphincter.

Pancreas

The pancreas, a long, thin gland extending from right to left across the abdomen, is divided into a head, body, and tail. The broader head lies close to the duodenum, the tail reaches the spleen on the left side. It is both an exocrine and an endocrine gland. The *exocrine* part of the gland produces pancreatic juice, which contains several important digestive enzymes. Pancreatic juice is emptied into the duodenum through the main pancreatic duct. The *endocrine* portion of the gland consists of scattered islets of Langerhans, which secrete the hormones insulin and glucagon directly into the blood stream.

Exocrine pancreas. The exocrine pancreas is a compound tubuloalveolar gland separated into lobules by loose connective tissue partitions (septa). These are continuous with a sheath of areolar connective tissue covering the entire organ. The glandular epithelium is composed of single-layer pyramidal serous cells that secrete a clear albuminous fluid containing enzymes. The cytoplasm is granular and stains darkly at the base of the cells. The cells are arranged in acini, or alveoli (Fig. 8-8). An acinus is a small grapelike sac, one of the secreting endpieces of a compound gland. (The words acinus and alveolus are used interchangeably when describing glandular structure.) The secretions of the acinar cells drain into small ducts, which in turn unite to form larger ducts. The pancreatic lobules are filled with many acini as well as small ducts, called intercalated ducts, which are composed of single-layer flattened cuboidal cells.

In the interlobular connective tissue, larger irregularly shaped collecting ducts lined with columnar or cuboidal cells can be seen.

Endocrine pancreas. In addition to the pancreatic acini, pancreatic lobules also contain scattered islands of cells known as the *islets of Langerhans* (Fig. 8-8). The islets are composed of cords of polyhedral pale-staining cells that can be easily differentiated from acinar cells. In and around the cords there is a rich capillary network. Although the islet cells closely resemble each other, special staining techniques can distinguish at least two types of cells, the alpha cells and the beta cells.

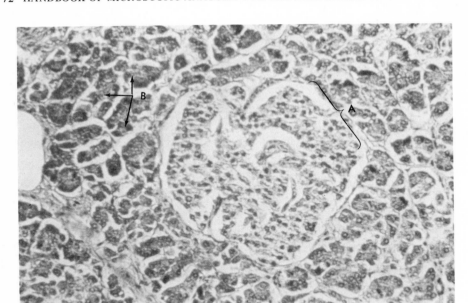

Fig. 8-8. Pancreas. *A*, Islet of Langerhans, *B*, pancreatic acini. (×100.)

Beta cells are more numerous and produce the hormone *insulin,* which controls carbohydrate metabolism in the body. A deficiency of this hormone causes diabetes mellitus. The *alpha cells* produce the hormone *glucagon,* which increases the level of glucose in the blood.

TUMORS OF THE LIVER AND THE PANCREAS
Primary cancer of the liver

Primary cancer of the liver is not a common disease. Secondary tumors of the liver that have metastasized from other organs are twenty-five times more frequently found than primary tumors. There are two types of primary carcinoma of the liver. The first type, seen in the majority of cases, is the malignant hepatoma that is derived from liver cells (Fig. 8-9). The second type is the malignant cholangioma, a glandular tumor arising from bile duct epithelium. Some liver tumors are composed of mixed cells of both types.

Histologically, hepatoma cells resemble normal liver cells. The malignant cells are arranged in solid columns, with some attempt at lobule formation. The cells are smaller than normal and stain more deeply. The nuclei are hyperchromatic, and many mitotic figures can be seen. Bile pigment is usually present in the cytoplasm. Cholangioma cells are low columnar or cuboidal in shape and show a tubular arrangement resembling that of normal bile ducts.

These tumors tend to invade the hepatic and portal veins and metastasize to the heart and lungs.

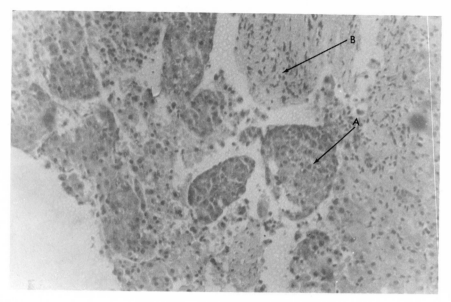

Fig. 8-9. Primary cancer of the liver. *A,* small dark-staining malignant hepatoma cells, *B,* fibrous stroma. (X100.)

Hepatoma is frequently correlated with *cirrhosis* of the liver, a condition characterized by destruction of liver cells and an increase in fibrous connective tissue in the liver. Although relatively rare in North America, hepatoma is rather frequently encountered in Africa and the Orient. The reasons for the high incidence of hepatoma in those areas has been the subject of much investigation in the last decade. It is now considered that fungal infections of the grains and nuts ingested by these populations may be, at least to some extent, the causative factor. Fungi growing on foods in moist tropical climates produce toxins that are known to damage the liver. One of these mycotoxins, aflatoxin, has been extracted from the fungus *Aspergillus,* which grows on peanuts. Aflatoxin produces severe liver damage, and also hepatomas, when fed to animals.

Cancer of the pancreas

Carcinoma of the pancreas is a relatively uncommon tumor involving the head of the gland more frequently than the tail. The growth can obstruct the common bile duct and cause an intense jaundice.

Three types of tumors, all adenocarcinomas, can occur in the pancreas: those arising from the simple columnar epithelium lining the ducts, those arising from the acinar cells, and endocrine tumors arising from the cells of the islets of Langerhans.

Adenocarcinomas originating from the duct epithelium are most often seen (Fig.

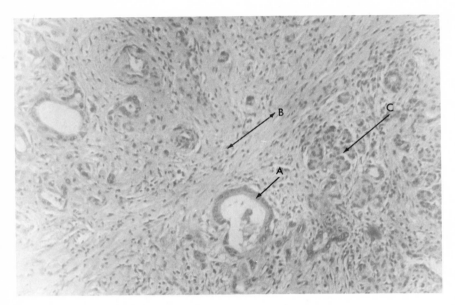

Fig. 8-10. Adenocarcinoma of the pancreas. *A*, Malignant cells forming atypical ducts, *B*, densely fibrous stroma, *C*, islet of Langerhans. (×100.)

8-10). The neoplastic cells are cuboidal or cylindrical in shape, and form irregular, atypical, dilated ducts. The malignant ducts are scattered in a very dense fibrous connective tissue stroma that obliterates most of the pancreatic acini. However, intact islets of Langerhans may still be seen in the connective tissue.

Tumors in the tail of the pancreas generally destroy many islet cells, and hyperglycemia may develop as a result.

The tumors spread by direct invasion of surrounding structures, for example, the duodenum, and colon, by invasion of lymphatics and regional lymph nodes, and through blood vessels to distant organs.

Functioning islet cell tumors (beta cell tumors) are usually accompanied by symptoms of marked hyperinsulinism.

9

Respiratory system

The respiratory system consists of a pair of lungs, which lie in the thorax, or chest cavity, and the passages that lead into the lungs from the outside. The general design of this system is that of a tree; the tree trunk is the single passage from the nose, through the pharynx, or throat, through the *larynx,* or voice box, into the *trachea,* or windpipe. Just as a tree trunk first divides into large branches, which then subdivide again and again into progressively smaller and more numerous branches, the trachea bifurcates (divides into two branches) into a right and left primary *bronchus,* each of which enters, respectively, the right and left lung at the hilus (a depression on the medial portion of the lung). Inside the substance of the lung, the primary bronchi subdivide into more numerous secondary bronchi, which in turn subdivide repeatedly into *bronchioles* (small bronchi). The smallest bronchioles finally terminate in the alveoli of the lungs, where the exchange of the respiratory gases, oxygen and carbon dioxide, takes place. In its passage from the outside into the lungs, the inspired air is warmed, moistened, and cleared of particulate material.

The histologic structure of the respiratory tract resembles, in general, that of other tubular passageways in the body. The innermost lining of the tube is a moist mucous membrane (mucosa), composed of epithelial cells resting on a basement membrane, and a lamina propria, composed of connective tissue immediately below the basement membrane. A second layer of connective tissue, the submucosa, lies below the lamina propria. Many mixed secreting glands can be found in this layer. Below the submucosa there may be a layer of muscle tissue, skeletal in some areas and smooth in others. The outermost coat, or tunica adventitia, is a fibrous connective tissue sheath.

Although the general architectural pattern is similar, there is some variation in structural detail at different levels of the respiratory tract.

NASAL CAVITY

The lining of the nasal cavity is initially continuous with the skin and is composed of stratified squamous epithelium with hair follicles, sebaceous glands, and sweat glands. This epithelium gradually loses its keratin and stratification and changes to a mucous membrane composed of ciliated, pseudostratified columnar cells, with numerous goblet cells, as the nasal passages move inward. A basement membrane and a lamina propria containing seromucous glands lie below the epithelium. Portions of the mucosa in the nasal cavity contain nerve cells that are receptors for the sense of smell. In these areas, bipolar neurons (olfactory cells) can be seen lying among the epithelial cells. The lamina propria in the nasal cavity is highly vascular and continuous with the periosteum (fibrous connective tissue sheath) that lies over the facial bones forming the cavity.

NASOPHARYNX

The nasal cavity leads into the nasopharynx, which has substantially the same structure, with the addition of a submucosal layer and a muscular tunic composed of skeletal muscle. The lamina contains aggregates of lymphoid tissue. On the posterior surface of the nasopharynx, there is an accumulation of lymphoid tissue forming the adenoids, or pharyngeal tonsil.

LARYNX

The larynx, or voice box, is a triangular boxlike structure connecting the nasopharynx with the trachea. Its walls are composed of nine cartilaginous plates and skeletal muscle. The larger cartilages are hyaline, the smaller ones are elastic cartilage. The inner lining is predominantly ciliated pseudostratified columnar epithelium, although the vocal cords and the uppermost cartilage of the larynx, the epiglottis, are covered with stratified squamous epithelium.

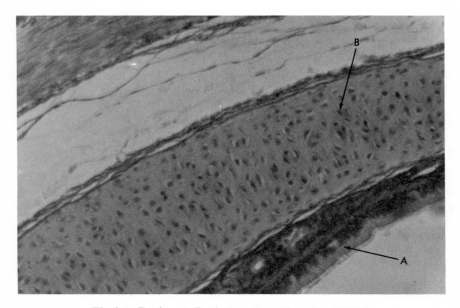

Fig. 9-1. Trachea. *A*, Epithelium, *B*, cartilage ring. (X100.)

The presence of cartilage in the walls of the larynx, the trachea, and the bronchi ensures that these passages will not collapse and obstruct the free flow of air into the lungs.

TRACHEA AND LARGER BRONCHI

The trachea and its larger branches are similar in structure. These tubes are lined with a mucosa consisting of ciliated pseudostratified columnar epithelium and many goblet cells (Fig. 9-1). A thick basement membrane separates these cells from the thin lamina propria, which contains white and elastic fibers. A submucosa, with seromucous glands, lies below the lamina. The adventitia of the trachea contains horseshoe-shaped rings of hyaline cartilage that open posteriorly on the surface facing the esophagus. The open area is filled with fibroelastic tissue and smooth muscle fibers.

SMALLER INTRAPULMONARY BRONCHI

As the bronchi in the lung subdivide into small tubes, the ciliated pseudostratified epithelium gradually changes to ciliated simple columnar epithelium containing some goblet cells. A muscularis mucosae, consisting of an increasing number of smooth muscle fibers, makes its appearance. The submucosa remains the same. The adventitia contains separate plates of hyaline cartilage, rather than rings, and these plates completely surround the tubes.

BRONCHIOLES

Respiratory tubes that are 1 mm in diameter or less are called bronchioles. Structural components present in the larger tubes undergo gradual changes. The epithelium is reduced from columnar to low cuboidal single-layer cells. Goblet cells disappear, as do the cartilage and glands. The walls are mainly composed of smooth muscle and elastic fibers. The smallest of these bronchioles, the terminal bronchioles, subdivide into respiratory bronchioles.

RESPIRATORY UNIT

Those portions of the respiratory system that are involved in the exchange of oxygen and carbon dioxide are known collectively as the respiratory unit. This includes the respiratory bronchioles, the alveolar ducts, and the alveoli.

Respiratory bronchioles are short, thin-walled tubules mainly lined by simple cuboidal epithelium. Cilia are sparse or not present. The wall is composed of collagenous and elastic fibers, with some smooth muscle fibers. A few alveoli open into the walls of these tubules at intervals, but the main mass of alveoli are in clusters, called alveolar sacs, that open into alveolar ducts. The histologic appearance of the alveolar sacs resembles a honeycomb, with each alveolus forming a separate cubicle opening into the lumen of the sac. Elastic and reticular fibers supply the supporting framework for these structures. The alveolar epithelium consists of a single layer of extremely thin, flattened cells, resting on a narrow basement membrane that adjoins the endothelium of the numerous pulmonary capillaries surrounding the alveoli. The total thickness of these three layers—the alveolar cells, the basement membrane, and the endothelial cells—is about 0.5 micron. It is here that the major exchange of respiratory gases between the blood and the air in the alveoli takes place. At intervals along the alveolar walls, pale vacuolated cells can be seen. These are believed to secrete a detergent substance, called *surfactant,* onto the alveolar surfaces, which prevents the collapse of the thin moist alveolar walls at each expiration. Also present are alveolar phagocytes, or *dust cells,* which engulf dust and smoke particles in inspired air, thus taking over the function of the ciliated cells of the larger air passages.

LUNGS AND PLEURAE

The right lung is divided into three lobes, the left lung into two. These lobes then divide into many hundreds of smaller lobules separated by thin connective tissue interlobular septa. The individual lobules contain a system of bronchi, bronchioles, and alveolar sacs (Fig. 9-2). Each lobule may therefore be considered a miniature lung in structure.

A pleural membrane lines the wall of the thoracic cavity (parietal pleura) and is reflected over each lung (visceral pleura). A potential space, filled with a small amount of pleural fluid, lies between the two pleurae. These are moist serous membranes, the exposed surfaces being covered by mesothelium, a type of simple squamous epithelium. The epithelium is supported by a lamina propria containing collagenous and elastic fibers, lymphatics, and a great number of blood vessels.

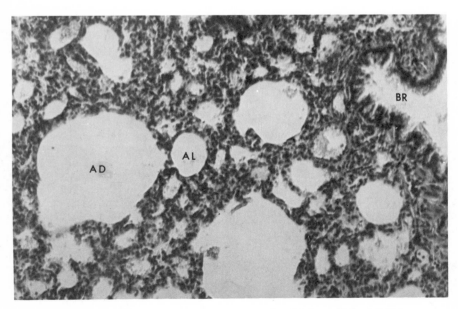

Fig. 9-2. Lung. *AD*, alveolar duct, *AL*, alveolus, *BR*, bronchiole. (X100.)

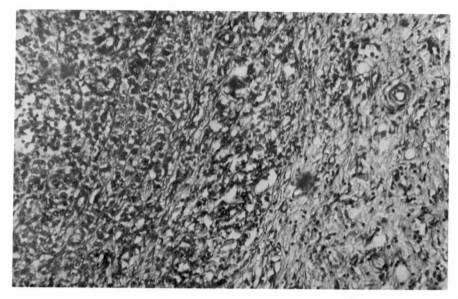

Fig. 9-3. Undifferentiated bronchogenic carcinoma. Malignant cells have replaced normal histologic structures of bronchus and surrounding lung. (×100.)

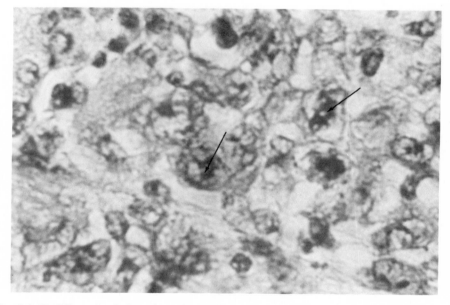

Fig. 9-4. Undifferentiated bronchogenic carcinoma. (×400.) Detail showing pleomorphism of tumor cells, mitotic figures (*arrows*).

CANCER OF THE LUNG (BRONCHOGENIC CARCINOMA)

Although any of the epithelial types in the respiratory tract may potentially become malignant, the most common epithelial tumor of the lung is a bronchogenic carcinoma (Fig. 9-3), arising usually at or near the bifurcation of the trachea into primary bronchi or in a major secondary bronchus. The right lung is more frequently involved than the left. The neoplastic cells are derived from bronchial epithelium, although they bear little resemblance to the normal ciliated columnar epithelium lining the bronchi. This characteristic property of tumor cells to assume different shapes and forms is called *pleomorphism* (Fig. 9-4). Bronchogenic carcinomas are often undifferentiated and can be composed of a mixture of cells: polygonal squamous-type cells, cuboidal cells, round cells, spindle-shaped "oat" cells, and bizarre giant cells. Columns of tumor cells erode the bronchial mucosa, invade the submucosa, and destroy the cartilage of the walls. Since the mass obstructs the lumen of a bronchus as it grows, pneumonia or pulmonary abscess tends to develop in the lung tissue distal to the obstruction. The tumor disseminates to distant areas of the body by invading the extensive lymphatic and vascular networks of the lung. Masses of neoplastic cells may also spread through the air spaces of the lung, from alveolus to alveolus.

The increasing incidence of bronchogenic carcinoma in the twentieth century has now been definitely linked to the inhalation of *carcinogenic hydrocarbons*, mainly in cigarette smoke. An additional hazard is the presence of these carcinogens in the atmosphere as a result of industrial pollution.

10

Urinary system

The urinary system consists of a right and left *kidney,* a right and left *ureter,* a single *urinary bladder,* and a single *urethra.* The ureters are tubes connecting the kidneys to the urinary bladder. The *urethra* is a passage connecting the urinary bladder to the exterior of the body. In the human male, the ejaculatory ducts merge with the urethra, which thus serves both as an excretory and reproductive outlet. In the human female, however, the urethra is separate from the genital system and serves only as an excretory duct.

The kidneys are bean-shaped organs with an indented slit, or hilus, on the medial surface, through which the ureters, blood vessels, lymphatics, and nerves pass into the substance of the kidney. Each human kidney is subdivided into an outer, dark red cortex, a lighter striated region called the medulla, and a funnel-shaped pelvis that lies in a shallow cavity called the *renal sinus.* The medulla is composed of about twelve cone-shaped structures, the *renal pyramids.* The broad base of each pyramid borders on the cortex, and the apex of each pyramid forms a nipple-shaped projection, or papilla, which extends into the renal sinus. Portions of the cortex dip down into the spaces between the pyramids, forming the renal columns. The *renal pelvis* is a fan-shaped expansion of the ureter. At its widest border, it forms two or three cuplike structures called the *major calyces,* which then subdivide into small *minor calyces.* Each minor calyx serves as a drain for the papilla of a pyramid. Urine flows from the pyramids, through the minor and major calyces, into the renal pelvis, then out of the kidneys and into the ureters.

NEPHRON

The kidney is a compound tubular gland composed of secretory tubules and collecting ducts. The substance that is secreted is a filtrate of blood. This filtrate is processed in the renal tubules and eventually excreted as urine. The functional unit of the kidney is called a *nephron.* There are about 1 million nephrons in each kidney. Each nephron consists of a *renal corpuscle,* a *proximal convoluted tubule, Henle's loop,* a *distal convoluted tubule,* and collecting tubules (excretory ducts). In general. the renal corpuscles, the proximal convoluted tubules, and most of the distal convoluted tubules are in the cortex of the kidney; Henle's loops and most of the collecting ducts are in the medullary pyramids of the kidney.

The renal corpuscle (Fig. 10-1) is an ultrafiltration device that can filter from the blood any soluble substance with a molecular weight of approximately less than 50,000. Since many of these substances are essential to the body, they are subsequently reabsorbed into the blood from the renal tubules.

Each renal corpuscle consists of a tuft of capillaries, called the *glomerulus,* and a double-walled cup-shaped structure surrounding the glomerulus, called *Bowman's capsule.*

The glomerulus is made up of four or five capillary loops, which branch off from an afferent arteriole and then merge and drain into a smaller efferent arteriole. Each renal corpuscle thus has its own afferent and efferent arteriole. The glomerular capillary wall is lined with simple squamous endothelium, as are all other capillaries in the body. However, this endothelium is extremely thin, with large pores that make it more permeable than other endothelia. A relatively thick glomerular basement membrane composed of collagen supports the endothelium.

Bowman's capsule is composed of a double layer of simple squamous epithelium. Its inner *visceral layer* is in close contact with the glomerulus, and its outer *parietal layer* is continuous with the neck of the proximal convoluted tubule.

The proximal convoluted tubule is composed of simple low columnar epithelial cells, with a prominent brush border *(microvilli)* facing the lumen of the tube. The

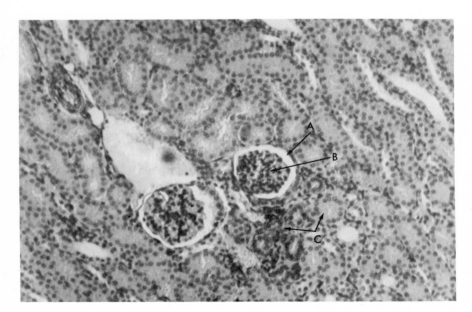

Fig. 10-1. Kidney. Renal cortex with renal corpuscles. *A,* Bowman's capsule, *B,* glomerulus, *C,* renal tubules. (×100.)

cells of the proximal convoluted tubule are very active in the reabsorption of water, electrolytes, amino acids, and glucose from the glomerular filtrate.

Henle's loop is a hairpin-shaped tubule with a descending segment, a thin U-shaped segment, and an ascending segment. The descending thick segment is a continuation of the epithelium of the proximal convoluted tubule. The thin segment of the loop is composed of pale-staining simple squamous epithelial cells with flattened nuclei. There are some microvilli, but no definite brush border. The ascending thick segment is the same as and continuous with the distal convoluted tubule. The loop system is responsible for the reabsorption of water from the glomerular filtrate and the formation of hypertonic urine.

The distal convoluted tubule has a wider lumen than the proximal convoluted tubule, and lacks a brush border. It is made up of simple low cuboidal epithelium, with a few microvilli. The distal convoluted tubule ascends into the cortex and runs close to the renal corpuscle from which it originated. At its closest point, where it runs next to the afferent and efferent arterioles supplying the renal corpuscle, the wall of the distal tubule has a special set of tall closely packed cells, the macula densa. These cells, together with specialized cells in the tunica media of the afferent arteriole, constitute the *juxtaglomerular apparatus,* which secretes a hormone called *renin.* Renin, in combination with a plasma globulin, forms *angiotensin,* a substance that raises the blood pressure.

The distal tubules empty into smaller collecting tubules, which then merge to form

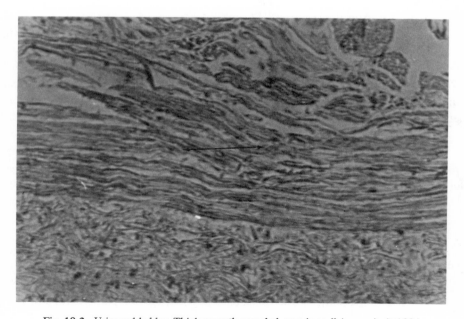

Fig. 10-2. Urinary bladder. Thick smooth muscle layers in wall (*arrows*). (X100.)

larger excretory ducts in the outer zone of the medulla. The larger ducts converge into even larger straight papillary ducts (the ducts of Bellini), which empty through the papillae of the pyramids into the minor calyces. Each papilla contains sixteen to twenty papillary ducts. The excretory duct walls are composed of regularly arranged simple cuboidal epithelium, which becomes taller and more columnar in shape as the ducts become larger. The cytoplasm of these cells is pale staining, and the nuclei are evenly arranged at the base of the cells.

RENAL PELVIS, URETER, AND URINARY BLADDER

The renal pelvis, ureter, and urinary bladder are hollow organs with similar histology. Their walls are composed of a mucosa consisting of specialized transitional epithelium, that rests on a lamina propria of collagenous connective tissue, a muscularis consisting of two to three layers of longitudinal and circular smooth muscle, and an adventitia made up of loose connective tissue. The three layers vary somewhat at different levels of the urinary tract: they are thinnest in the renal pelvis and thickest in the urinary bladder. The lower portion of each ureter and the urinary bladder have a thick three-layered muscularis. In the bladder (Fig. 10-2), the smooth muscle is arranged in a circular sphincter around the urethral opening. The upper surface of the bladder is covered with peritoneum, and thus has a serosa rather than an adventitia.

URETHRA

The urethra is the duct that connects the urinary bladder to the exterior of the body. Its wall is generally composed of three layers: a mucosa, a muscularis, and an adventitia. There is variation in the composition of these layers, as well as differences in the structural anatomy of the female and male urethras.

The urethra of the female is a short tube about 3 cm long. The lumen is a narrow folded crescent, lined by transitional epithelium closest to the bladder and mixed pseudostratified columnar and stratified squamous epithelium farther from the bladder. Small groups of mucus-secreting cells are present in the epithelium. The lamina propria is a wide band of connective tissue containing elastic fibers and a plexus of thin-walled veins, which give it the appearance of a corpus spongiosum. The muscularis is composed of a double layer of longitudinal and circular smooth muscle fibers. At the lower end of the urethra, the circular smooth muscle is reinforced by skeletal muscle fibers that form the voluntary constrictor muscle of the urethral sphincter.

The male urethra is about 20 cm long and consists of three distinct segments.

The *prostatic urethra* extends from the urinary bladder through the prostate gland. It is about 3 or 4 cm long and is lined by transitional epithelium. The lamina propria and muscularis resemble that of the female urethra. The circular smooth muscle is continuous with the smooth muscle sphincter at the neck of the bladder. The prostatic urethra is surrounded by the prostate gland, from which it receives numerous ducts.

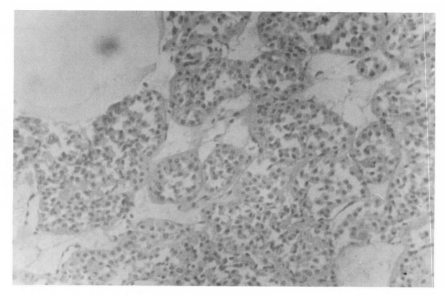

Fig. 10-3. Renal cell carcinoma. Malignant cuboidal cells forming tubular structures. (×100.)

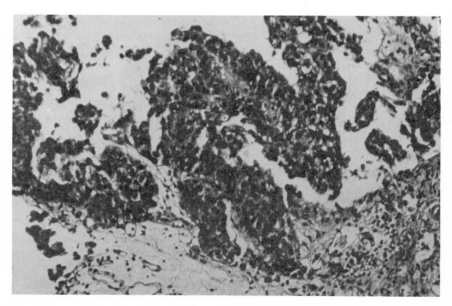

Fig. 10-4. Transitional cell carcinoma of the urinary bladder. Thickened epithelium with atypical cells invading tissues of the bladder wall. (×100.)

The two ejaculatory ducts of the male reproductive tract also empty into the prostatic urethra.

The *membranous urethra* is a short segment that extends from just below the prostate gland to the root of the penis. It is lined by pseudostratified and stratified columnar epithelium. The smooth muscle of the membranous urethra is surrounded by striated muscle fibers that form the voluntary external sphincter of the male urinary tract.

The *cavernous urethra,* or spongy urethra, is about 15 cm long and extends from the root of the penis to the glans penis. The epithelial lining is mainly pseudostratified columnar epithelium, which changes gradually to stratified squamous epithelium at the glans. The lamina propria is part of the erectile tissue of the corpus spongiosum, which surrounds the cavernous urethra. The mucus-secreting glands in the lamina are most numerous in the cavernous urethra, although they occur in the prostatic and membranous urethra as well. There is no distinct muscularis layer, but some scattered bundles of smooth muscle fibers are present.

MALIGNANT TUMORS OF THE URINARY TRACT
Adenocarcinoma of the kidney (renal cell carcinoma, hypernephroma)

Most tumors in the kidney originate in the cortex and arise from the epithelium of the convoluted tubules (Fig. 10-3). They are relatively uncommon. The cells usually show much variation in histologic appearance. They may be tall columnar, cuboidal, or spindle shaped. The cytoplasm may be clear, foamy, and light-staining, with small round nuclei, or granular and eosinophilic, with large dark-staining nuclei. Very often, both clear cells and granular cells are present in the same tumor. Acinar or tubular structures may predominate, or the tumor cells may form solid sheets.

Renal tumors metastasize to distant organs by way of the regional lymph nodes and also through the renal vein.

Carcinoma of the urinary bladder

Transitional cell carcinomas arise from the transitional epithelium that composes the mucosal lining of the bladder (Fig. 10-4). The malignant epithelial cells vary markedly in size and shape. They appear polygonal or spherical, with hyperchromatic nuclei. Giant cells and bizarre cell forms are frequently seen. The epithelial layers are thicker, and the normal arrangement of basal cells on a basement membrane is not seen. Masses of dark-staining, rapidly proliferating malignant cells may invade the smooth muscle wall of the bladder.

The tumor can metastasize by way of the lymph nodes and also invades neighboring pelvic organs by direct spread. A common complication is the development of infections of the renal pelvis (pyelonephritis).

There is a high incidence of this tumor in workers in dye factories, particularly those exposed for many years to the compound betanaphthylamine. It may also develop following schistosomiasis, a parasitic disease common in Africa.

11

Female reproductive system

The female reproductive system consists of a pair of ovaries, a pair of oviducts (Fallopian tubes), a uterus, a vagina, and external genitalia.

OVARIES

The ovaries are small glands lying on either side of the uterus in the pelvic cavity. They are attached to the broad ligament of the uterus by a double fold of peritoneum and to the pelvic wall by suspensory ligaments.

These glands have both exocrine and endocrine functions; that is, they secrete *ova* (egg cells) into a duct (the Fallopian tube), and they secrete the female sex hormones, *estrogen* and *progesterone,* directly into the blood stream.

The free surface of the ovaries is covered with a layer of simple cuboidal to columnar epithelium. This layer is also called the *germinal epithelium,* because it is considered by some to be the source of the primitive egg cells in the fetal ovary. Beneath the epithelium is a layer of dense connective tissue called the *tunica albuginea.*

The interior of the ovary consists of a medulla and a cortex, although the boundary between these two zones is not sharp. The central inner core, the medulla, is made up of loose connective tissue containing many nerves, lymphatics, and blood vessels, which enter the ovary at the hilus, a small depression on the surface of the ovary. The cortex, or outer shell of the gland, is composed of a rather unusual connective tissue stroma (or supporting framework), with large spindle-shaped cells that resemble the primitive fibroblasts found in embryonal tissues. A thin mesh of reticular fibers fills the spaces between these cells. Embedded in the stroma are *follicles* (small sacs) in various stages of development (Figs. 11-1 and 11-2). Each contains an *ovum* (egg cell). From time to time, after puberty, a follicle and its ovum will enlarge and move toward the surface of the ovary. If its development continues, the follicle will eventually form a blisterlike structure on the surface of the ovary, then rupture and release the ovum into the Fallopian tube.

At birth, a female has about 400,000 primary follicles, each containing a primitive ovum, scattered in the cortex of the ovaries. The majority of these follicles degenerate,

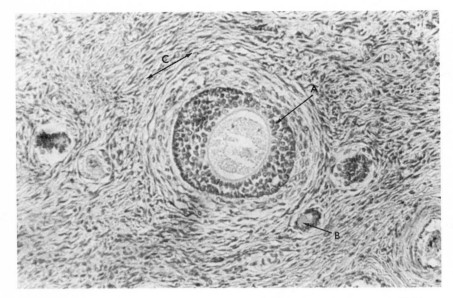

Fig. 11-1. Ovary. *A*, Growing follicle, *B*, atretic follicle, *C*, ovarian stroma. (X100.)

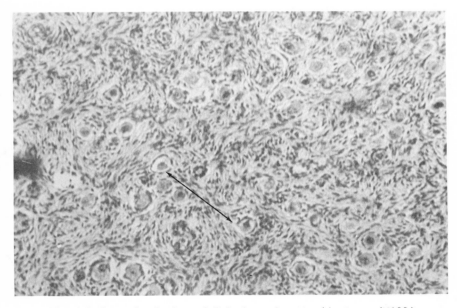

Fig. 11-2. Ovary. Small primary follicles (*arrows*) scattered in stroma. (X100.)

or undergo atresia; the surviving follicles remain. After puberty, one ovum is released approximately every 4 weeks, in the cyclic process known as ovulation. This pattern continues until menopause, the cessation of the menstrual and reproductive cycles in women.

Growth and development of follicles

The primary follicle consists of a single layer of squamous epithelial cells called follicle cells. In the center of the follicle is the large round ovum.

During the growth phase, the ovum and the follicle increase in size. The squamous cells that made up the primary follicle become first cuboidal and then stratified columnar, thickening on one side and thus making the follicle oval in shape. Yolk granules appear in the ovum. The enlarged follicle then hollows out and develops spaces filled with fluid *(liquor folliculi)*. The follicle is now called a *Graafian follicle.*

The connective tissue stroma around the follicle forms a two-layered capsule. The inner layer is called the theca interna. It is separated from the follicle cells by a basement membrane. The outer layer is a dense fibrous connective tissue layer called the theca externa.

As the Graafian follicle enlarges, it gradually pushes to the surface of the ovary. The production of Graafian follicles in the ovary is initiated by the *follicle-stimulating hormone* (FSH) secreted by the anterior lobe of the pituitary gland *(adenohypophysis)*. When the Graafian follicle is fully developed, it will either rupture and release the ovum *(ovulation)* or involute *(undergo atresia)* (Fig. 11-1).

Just prior to ovulation, the first maturation division occurs in the ovum. It divides by meiosis, and the number of chromosomes is halved (in the human germ cell, half the number of chromosomes, or *haploid number,* is 23). One daughter cell, the *oocyte,* and one small nonfunctioning *polar body* are produced by this division.

During their development, the follicle cells produce the hormone *estrogen,* which is responsible for the growth and development of secondary sex characteristics, stimulation of the lining *(endometrium)* of the uterus, and stimulation of mammary growth.

After the Graafian follicle has ruptured and the ovum is released, a glandular structure called the *corpus luteum* (yellow body) forms in the remnant of the follicle. The lining cells change their appearance and become lutein cells. Some of the theca interna cells also transform to lutein cells. The corpus luteum produces the hormone *progesterone,* which prepares the uterine endometrium for the implantation of the fertilized ovum and also stimulates growth of the mammary glands. If pregnancy occurs, the corpus luteum persists throughout pregnancy. If pregnancy does not occur, the corpus luteum gradually involutes (ceases to produce progesterone) and forms a white scar known as the *corpus albicans* (white body).

During the reproductive years, ovarian follicles can be seen in all stages of development and involution.

FALLOPIAN TUBES

The Fallopian tubes, or *oviducts,* are muscular tubes about 4½ inches long, that extend from the ovaries to the uterus. They are continuous with the uterus at its upper portion. They are not directly connected with the ovaries, but have a funnel-shaped opening over each ovary, which is split into *fimbria,* or fringes.

The wall of an oviduct is composed of an extensively folded mucous membrane made up of simple or pseudostratified columnar epithelium, taller and ciliated at the ovarian end and gradually becoming shorter and nonciliated as the tube approaches the uterus. The epithelium rests on a lamina propria made up of many spindle-shaped connective tissue cells and a few collagenous fibers. There is no submucosa. The mucous membrane is surrounded by two layers of smooth muscle, an inner circular layer and an outer longitudinal layer. The outermost coat is a serosa, which is part of the peritoneum.

The fimbriated ends of the Fallopian tubes receive the ovum after the rupture of the Graafian follicle. The ovum is propelled toward the uterus by the cilia of the epithelial lining of the oviducts and possibly by contraction of the smooth muscle of the wall. Fertilization of the ovum by the male sperm cell takes place in the Fallopian tube. After 2 or 3 days, the fertilized ovum reaches the uterine lumen, where it implants itself in the endometrium.

UTERUS

The uterus is a hollow, pear-shaped organ lying in the pelvic cavity between the urinary bladder and the sigmoid colon and rectum. The main expanded portion of the uterus is called the *body;* the narrower neck at its lower end, which opens into the vagina, is called the *cervix.* The dome-shaped upper portion of the uterus, the *fundus,* is continuous with the oviducts (Fallopian tubes).

The function of the uterus is to house, protect, and nourish the developing embryo and to expel it when the period of gestation is concluded.

The wall of the uterus consists of an inner mucosa called the *endometrium,* a smooth-muscle muscularis called the *myometrium,* and an outer serosa called the *perimetrium.* (The suffix -metrium is derived from the Greek *metra,* meaning womb.)

Endometrium

The surface of the endometrium consists of simple columnar epithelium, some of which is ciliated. These cells lie on a wide lamina propria, also called the endometrial stroma. The connective tissue stromal cells are stellate, with large ovoid nuclei. Reticular fibers supply the framework of the lamina. Granular leukocytes and lymphocytes can also be seen here. Extending through the full thickness of the lamina are long, simple tubular glands lined by simple columnar epithelium identical to that on the surface. These glands secrete mucus. The endometrium also contains specialized blood vessels, the coiled arteries, that extend high up into the lamina propria.

At intervals during the active reproductive life of the human female, the endometrium undergoes marked changes in appearance. These changes occur rhythmically in a monthly cycle, the menstrual cycle; they are associated with the ebb and flow of secretion of the ovarian hormones.

Four phases can be demonstrated in the endometrium during the cycle:

1. The *follicular phase (proliferative phase)* (Fig. 11-3) takes place during the formation of the Graafian follicle and is dependent upon estrogen. The endometrial lining is regenerated following the previous menstrual phase. The mucosa increases in thickness, the glands increase in number, and the connective tissue cells multiply and rebuild the lamina propria. This phase continues to day 13 or 14 of the cycle.

2. The *secretory phase (luteal phase, progestational phase)* (Fig. 11-4) starts about 14 days before the onset of menstruation (bleeding). The endometrium increases greatly in thickness due to an accumulation of tissue fluid. The glands secrete a thick mucoid substance containing glycogen. The coiled arteries extend nearly to the surface. If fertilization of the ovum occurs, the secretory phase persists and provides a bed for the implantation of the ovum. This phase is dependent on the secretion of the corpus luteal hormone, progesterone.

3. The *ischemic phase (premenstrual phase)* is associated with the constriction of the coiled arteries, which cuts off the blood supply to the enlarged portion of the endometrium. The cells become pale and shrunken, and there is a loss of fluid. This stage lasts for 1 or 2 days and ends with the first signs of external bleeding. This phase occurs as the corpus luteum involutes and the level of ovarian hormones drops.

4. During the *menstrual phase,* the upper three quarters of the endometrium sloughs off, tearing away glands, arteries, and veins. Pools of blood, which do not coagulate, collect in the lamina propria. A discharge consisting of blood, epithelial and stromal cells, and mucus leaves the reproductive tract by way of the vagina.

Myometrium

The middle layer of the uterus, the muscular layer, lies immediately below the lamina propria of the mucosa. It is a thick layer of interwoven bundles of large smooth muscle cells, which are separated by connective tissue. The myometrium composes about three fourths of the total thickness of the uterine wall. During pregancy, these smooth muscle cells increase greatly in number and size.

Perimetrium

The outermost serous membrane surrounding most of the uterus (and the oviducts) is an extension of the peritoneum. Like all other serous membranes of the body, the perimetrium is composed of specialized simple squamous epithelium, called mesothelium, with an underlying lamina composed usually of loose areolar connective tissue.

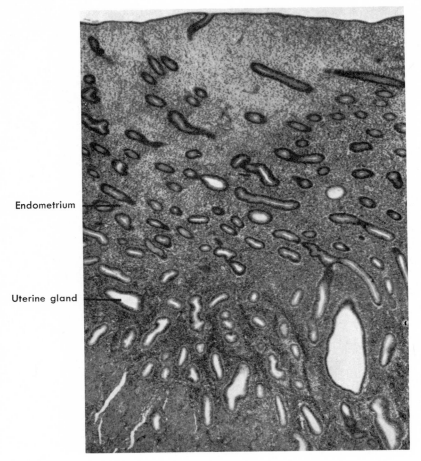

Endometrium

Uterine gland

Fig. 11-3. Follicular phase (proliferative phase) endometrium, human uterus. (X40.) Increased thickness of the mucosa and proliferation of the uterine glands. (From Bevelander-Ramaley: Essentials of histology, St. Louis, 1974, The C. V. Mosby Co.)

Cervix

The lining epithelium of the cervix is the same as that of the body of the uterus, but the cervical glands are highly branched. The lamina propria is less cellular and contains more fibers. The mucosa of the cervix is extensively and deeply folded. The cervical glands undergo slight changes during the menstrual cycle, but the cervical mucosa is not sloughed during menstruation. The lumen of the cervix, the cervical canal, is usually filled with a mucous plug. The outer wall of the cervix, which protrudes into the vagina, is covered by a continuation of the vaginal epithelium, thick stratified squamous unkeratinized epithelium.

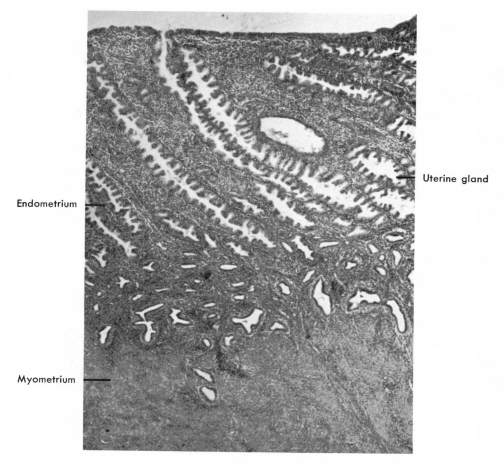

Endometrium

Myometrium

Uterine gland

Fig. 11-4. Secretory phase endometrium, human uterus. (×40.) Enlargement and sacculation of the uterine glands. (From Bevelander-Ramaley: Essentials of histology, St. Louis, 1974, The C. V. Mosby Co.)

VAGINA

The vagina is a tube about 3½ inches long. It is continous with the cervix at its upper end, and has a fold of mucosa, the hymen, at the vaginal orifice, or opening at the lower end.

The wall of the vagina consists of a mucosa and a submucosa, which are fused together, a muscularis, and an outer adventitia.

The mucosa is lined by thick, nonkeratinized stratified squamous epithelium resembling the epidermis of skin. The base of the epithelial layer is wavy and arranged in tall nipplelike ridges, or papillae. The lamina propria is composed of dense fibrous connective tissue and contains many blood vessels, some lymphoid tissue, and some elastic fibers. The mucosa is extensively folded. There are no glands, and lubricating mucus is supplied by the glands of the cervix.

The muscularis layer is composed of interlacing bundles of smooth-muscle fibers, some in circular, and some in longitudinal arrangements. At the vaginal orifice, there is a sphincter (circular ring) muscle composed of skeletal muscle.

The adventitia is made up of a thin layer of dense connectiv issue rich in blood vessels.

EXTERNAL GENITALIA

The external genitalia, the *vulva,* are bounded at the sides by the *labia majora* (greater lips), within which are the *labia minora* (lesser lips). The remainder of the vulva is a small area known as the *vestibule,* lying between the labia minora, which contains the *clitoris* and the openings of the urethra and the vagina.

The clitoris is analogous to the penis in the male, although it is small and rudimentary. It is composed of a central core of vascular erectile tissue, resembling the corpora cavernosa of the penis, and is covered with thin stratified squamous epithelium. The structure contains many specialized nerve endings such as *Meissner's corpuscles* (touch receptors), *Pacinian corpuscles* (pressure receptors), and *Krause's end bulbs* (temperature receptors).

The labia minora are thin folds of mucosa covered with stratified squamous epithelium containing sebaceous glands.

The labia majora are thicker folds composed of mucous membrane on the inner surface, and skin containing hair follicles, sweat glands, and sebaceous glands on the outer surface.

The vestibule is lubricated by tubuloalveolar glands that secrete mucus onto the surface. The largest of these glands are the paired *glands of Bartholin,* whose ducts open into the vestibule just outside the hymen.

TUMORS OF THE FEMALE REPRODUCTIVE SYSTEM
Carcinoma of the ovary

Cancer of the ovary occurs more frequently in women who are past the age of menopause. About one in every ten growths in the ovary is malignant.

The origin of many of the structural elements of the ovary is still in doubt, and there is some controversy about the classification of tumor types occurring in the ovary. One of the more common tumors found here is the *cystadenoma* (Fig. 11-5). The epithelium of this type of tumor secretes a serous fluid, and the tumor is cystic in nature. Cystadenoma may be obviously benign, or it may show areas of epithelial proliferation that are questionably malignant. Where the epithelium is frankly atypical and shows anaplasia (loss of normal architecture), a diagnosis of cystadenocarcinoma can be made. The proliferating cells are usually low cuboidal epithelial elements, with large hyperchromatic elongated nuclei. These cells are often arranged in papillae

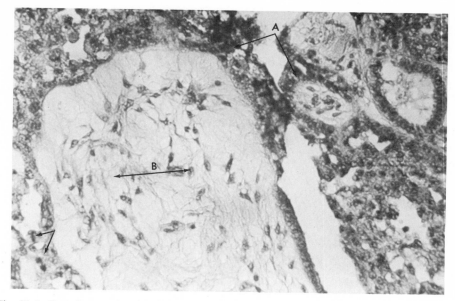

Fig. 11-5. Cystadenocarcinoma of the ovary. *A*, Malignant cuboidal cells; mitotic figures *(arrows)*, *B*, central core of connective tissue (ovarian stroma). (×100.)

(ridges) or alveoli (saclike glandular structures). The epithelium may enclose a central core of connective tissue stroma with sarcomalike features. The connective tissue stroma of the ovary is not merely a supporting tissue, but a functioning part of the ovarian parenchyma. It can undergo neoplastic changes together with the epithelial elements.

The tumor usually metastasizes to distant organs by way of lymphatics, and locally to the peritoneum.

Tumors of the uterus

Leiomyoma. This benign tumor is commonly known as "fibroids," although *leiomyoma* is a more accurate name (Gr. *leios,* smooth; Gr. *mys,* muscle) because it arises in the smooth muscle layer of the uterus, the myometrium (Fig. 11-6). It is the commonest tumor found in the female pelvis and tends to occur more frequently before menopause.

The leiomyoma is composed of the same types of tissue as the myometrium, namely, smooth muscle, connective tissue, blood vessels, and lymphatics. It may be considered a localized *hyperplasia* (an increase or overgrowth of the number of normal cells in a tissue), and is possibly caused by endocrine imbalance. The growths may be single or multiple and can occur just beneath the peritoneal covering of the uterus *(subserous fibroids),* in the wall of the uterus *(intramural fibroids),* or just below the mucosa *(submucous fibroids).* Leiomyomas are usually completely surrounded by a connective tissue capsule.

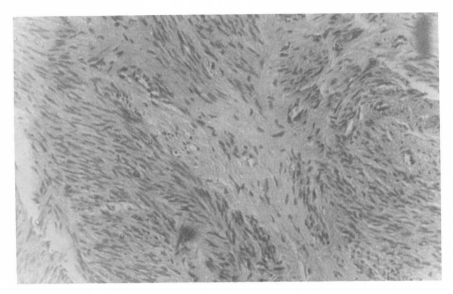

Fig. 11-6. Leiomyoma of the uterus. Benign tumor composed entirely of bundles of smooth muscle and fibrous connective tissue. (X100.)

Very often the tumors are asymptomatic and do not require treatment. However, submucous fibroids may bulge into the uterine cavity and cause abnormal bleeding, hemorrhage, and anemia. Large fibroids may also interfere with the functioning of the urinary bladder and the colon. In such instances, surgical removal of the uterus *(hysterectomy)* is the treatment of choice.

Carcinoma of the body of the uterus (endometrial carcinoma). The cavity of the uterus is lined throughout by simple columnar epithelium, which forms narrow tubular glands that extend deep into the endometrial stroma. The epithelial tissue is active and changes markedly during the phases of the menstrual cycle. At menopause, when the endocrine activity of the ovaries diminishes, the function of the endometrium ceases. The mucosa atrophies (wastes away), the glands become smaller and may disappear, and the stroma thins out. It is during this period that cancers of the body of the uterus frequently develop.

The typical architecture of a malignant endometrial tumor is that of a columnar cell adenocarcinoma (Fig. 11-7). There may be varying degrees of differentiation, that is, the malignant tissue sometimes forms glandular structures. Or the cells can be arranged as solid masses of proliferating columnar elements, large and small, showing many mitotic figures. A stroma is absent or scanty.

The tumor may locally invade the myometrium, serosa, peritoneum, cervix, and Fallopian tubes. Lymphatic and blood-borne metastases to distant organs also occur. The prognosis (prospect of cure) of this tumor is good when it is treated in the early stages by combined surgery and radiotherapy.

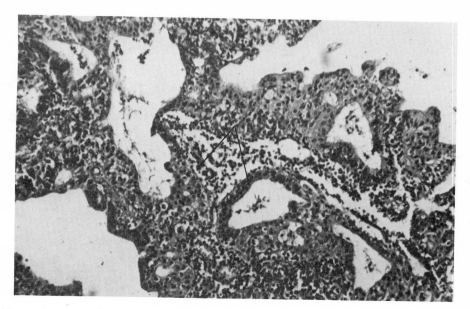

Fig. 11-7. Carcinoma of the uterine endometrium. Arrows indicate proliferating malignant columnar cells, some forming glands. (×100.)

Carcinoma of the cervix. Carcinoma of the cervix is second to cancer of the breast in its frequency. Its occurrence appears to be correlated with age at first sexual intercourse, frequency of sexual intercourse, and age at first pregnancy.

Most tumors of the cervix are epidermoid, squamous cell tumors arising from the outer mucosa of the cervix. The tumors can originate in any layer of the stratified squamous epithelium, that is, from germinal cells, basal cells, or cells of the intermediate layers. The tumor cells are cuboidal or polygonal in shape and usually grow in solid sheets. Many pleomorphic cells (cells of different shapes) can be seen. There is a loss of stratification, and an invasion of the underlying stroma (Figs. 11-8 and 11-9).

Radiotherapy is the treatment of choice in the early stages and results in a substantial cure rate. Carcinoma of the cervix lends itself to early detection by the Papanicolaou test, and periodic cytologic screening for this tumor has become routine in many clinics.

Papanicolaou test

This technique, described by Papanicolaou in 1942, consists of a series of nuclear and cytoplasmic stains adapted for the study of smears of cells that are normally shed or desquamated into various body cavities and tubes *(exfoliative cytology,* the study of individual cells that have been shed from a tissue). The test is used for the rapid

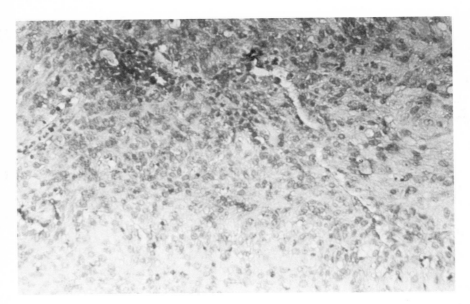

Fig. 11-8. Epidermoid carcinoma of the cervix. Sheets of malignant cells showing variation in nuclear size and shape. (×100.)

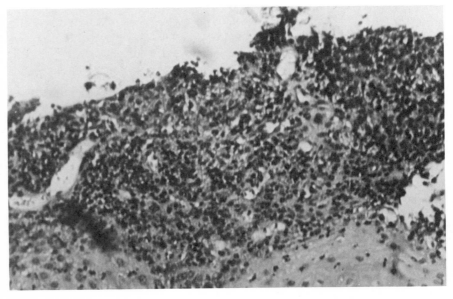

Fig. 11-9. Epidermoid carcinoma of the cervix. Area showing infection. Massed small dark cells are leukocytes. (×100.)

diagnosis of malignant cells desquamated into vaginal secretions, prostatic secretions, gastric juice, serous fluids in the body cavities, sputum, and urine. A diagnosis of malignancy made by this method must be checked by surgical removal of a small piece of the suspect area *(biopsy)* and the examination of routine histologic sections of the piece of tissue.

Criteria for malignancy are based on the appearance of the nuclei of malignant cells. These show certain features that are not seen in normal cells:

1. The nuclei stain darkly, and clumping of the chromatin is common. The borders of the malignant nuclei are usually sharply outlined by the stains.
2. Changes in the cytoplasmic/nuclear ratio are marked. Malignant nuclei are much larger than normal and occupy most of the cell. Usually, cytoplasm is not even visible. In addition, there is much variation in size among malignant nuclei. The malignant nucleus often presents a crinkled *(crenated)* appearance.

Smears are usually reported as positive, negative, or doubtful. Positive smears contain malignant cells, negative smears show only normal cells, and doubtful smears indicate the presence of isolated suspicious cells that are either *dyskaryotic* (contain peculiar nuclei) or *metaplastic* (a change to a type of cell that is not normally found in that tissue). Papanicolaou originally suggested a more elaborate system of classification, ranging from Class I to Class V. Briefly, Class I is negative, Classes II and III are doubtful, and Classes IV and V are positive.

Cytologic examination of cells shed from the uterine cervix may reveal the presence of small, easily curable tumors.

Most tumors of the cervix are squamous carcinomas originating from the stratified squamous epithelium of the mucosa. This highly stratified tissue is composed of four fairly well-defined layers: the deepest layer is the germinal layer, the layer above it is the basal layer, the third layer is the intermediate layer, and the uppermost layer is the superficial layer. The actively growing cells are found in the germinal layer. Germinal cells have a large nucleus and very little cytoplasm. As these cells mature and push up toward the surface, their morphology changes. There is an increase in the amount of cytoplasm and a decrease in nuclear size. The basal cells are oval or round, with a definite ring of cytoplasm and a large nucleus. The intermediate cells are identifiable as squamous cells, having an increased amount of cytoplasm with definite corners and nuclei very much reduced in size. The superficial cells are typical large, flat, polygonal squamous cells, with small dense, dark-staining *(pyknotic)* nuclei.

The finding of only superficial and intermediate cells on a vaginal smear is reported as negative. If there are many inner layer basal cells in the specimen, the smear is considered doubtful. When many cells with immature nuclei from the germinal layer are seen together with atypical cells, or when numbers of undifferentiated malignant cells are seen, the report is positive (Figs. 11-10 to 11-13).

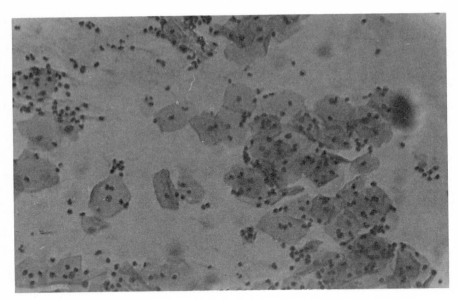

Fig. 11-10. Papanicolaou stain, normal cervical epithelium. Superficial and intermediate layer cells with small nuclei and large amount of cytoplasm. The cells are flat, and some have folded cytoplasm. Small dark cells are leukocytes. (X100.)

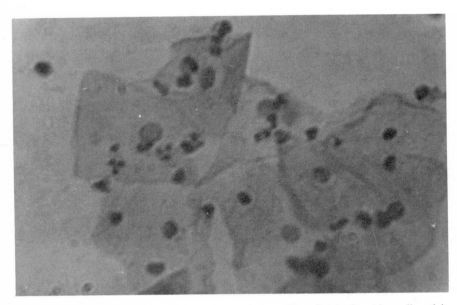

Fig. 11-11. Papanicolaou stain, normal cervical epithelium. Superficial cells with small nuclei, and intermediate layer cells with larger nuclei. Thin transparent cytoplasm may be folded over or wrinkled. (X400.)

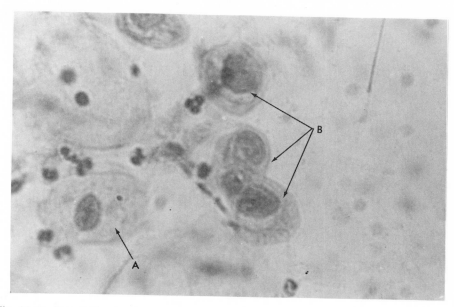

Fig. 11-12. Papanicolaou stain, cervical cells from basal layers. Round or oval cells with central nuclei containing fine granular chromatin. Amount and density of cytoplasm indicates maturity of cell. *A,* More mature basal cell from outer layers, *B,* inner basal cells. (X400.)

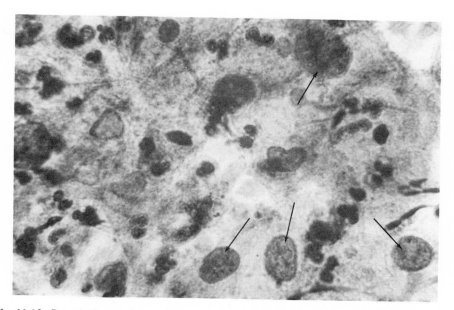

Fig. 11-13. Papanicolaou stain, carcinoma of the cervix. Cytoplasm of undifferentiated malignant cells (*arrows*) appears absent; large nuclei with sharp borders and clumped chromatin, showing marked variation in size and shape. (X400.)

THE MAMMARY GLAND

The mammary gland is a modified sweat gland. It is undeveloped in children and remains rudimentary in men. It enlarges in women after puberty, but only reaches full development during pregnancy and lactation.

The general structure of a developed mammary gland is that of a compound alveolar gland. The secreting epithelial cells and their small ducts are arranged in groups in a loose connective tissue bed. This constitutes a lobule (a small lobe). Dense fibrous connective tissue separates the lobules from each other. Larger ducts, the interlobular ducts, can be seen in the interlobular dense connective tissue. The lobules are in turn arranged into some fifteen to twenty larger lobes, each of which has its own excretory duct, the *lactiferous duct.* Each lactiferous duct has its separate opening into a projection on the surface of the breast, the nipple. A circular pigmented area on the skin, the *areola,* surrounds each nipple.

The glandular epithelium within the lobules is subject to hormonal control and shows marked differences in quantity and distribution, depending on whether the gland is in an inactive state, whether it is enlarging in preparation for lactation, or whether it is actively secreting milk.

The inactive gland

When the mammary gland is in the inactive state, the lobules are small and contain much loose connective tissue, with fine collagenous fibers and fibroblasts. Small intralobular ducts lined with simple cuboidal epithelium are scattered in the connective tissue. Alveoli as such (the spherical endpieces of the ducts) are barely recognizable or not present. The interlobular connective tissue (between the lobules) is abundant and dense, and contains many adipose cells. Larger interlobular ducts can be seen here, lined by a double layer columnar epithelium. In the main lactiferous ducts, the columnar epithelium becomes stratified. This is replaced by stratified squamous epithelium near the opening on the nipple. Branched myoepithelial basket cells, which are capable of contraction, can be seen between the epithelium and the underlying basement membrane of the ducts.

The gland during pregnancy

During pregnancy, the alveoli and interlobular secretory ducts, lined by simple cuboidal epithelium, proliferate rapidly. It is believed that estrogen is responsible for the growth of the ducts, and progesterone and estrogen jointly are responsible for the growth of the alveoli. The secretion of these two female sex hormones during the first half of pregnancy is greatly increased. The glandular epithelial structures expand into the intralobular connective tissue. As the lobules enlarge and become well defined, the interlobular septa become narrower and fat cells disappear.

The gland during lactation

During lactation, the alveoli enlarge and occupy most of the breast tissue (Fig. 11-14). The connective tissue elements are greatly reduced. Many alveoli are dilated,

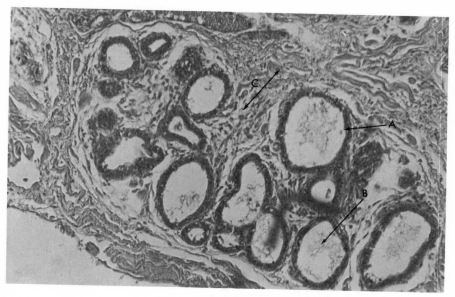

Fig. 11-14. Lactating mammary gland. *A*, Alveolus, *B*, milk, *C*, intralobular connective tissue. (X100.)

becoming saccules (small sacs) filled with milk. They are lined with cuboidal to columnar epithelium, and myoepithelial cells are present beneath the epithelium. Large fat droplets and protein granules can be seen in the glandular epithelium. The larger excretory ducts do not change appreciably during pregnancy and lactation.

Endocrine control of lactation and milk ejection

Lactation results after *parturition* (birth) as a result of the secretion of *lactogenic hormone, prolactin,* from the anterior lobe of the pituitary gland. This hormone cannot induce lactation unless the mammary gland has been prepared (the epithelial elements have proliferated extensively) by the action of estrogen and progesterone. Prolactin is not secreted until the level of these ovarian hormones drops sharply, as it does at parturition. Prolactin acts directly on the alveolar epithelium to stimulate the synthesis of the milky secretion.

The actual ejection of milk from the ducts and the alveoli is initiated by the sucking of the newborn infant. Afferent nerve endings in the nipple are stimulated and relay stimulation to the *hypothalamus,* bringing about a secretion of the hormone *oxytocin* from the posterior lobe of the pituitary gland *(neurohypophysis).* This hormone causes contraction of the myoepithelial cells of the ducts. The milk is then squeezed out of the smaller ducts to larger interlobular ducts. These in turn join and empty into the lactiferous ducts. Milk passes from these ducts into the nipple.

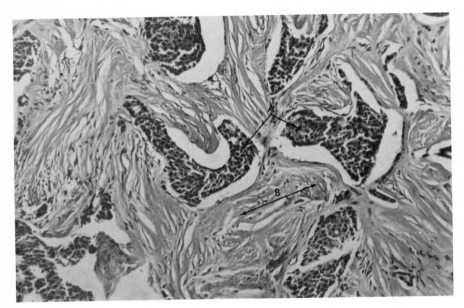

Fig. 11-15. Carcinoma of the breast. *A*, Strands of malignant cells, *B*, dense fibrous stroma. (×100.)

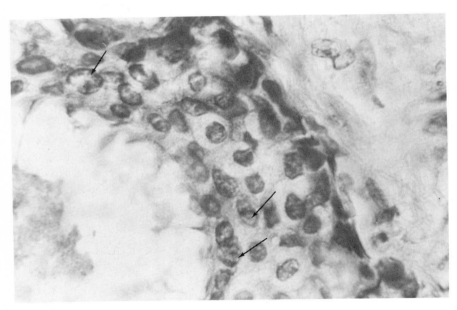

Fig. 11-16. Higher magnification of Fig. 11-15. (×400.) Small cuboidal malignant cells with mitotic figures (*arrows*).

Adenocarcinoma of the breast

Mammary cancer is the most common tumor in women over the age of 40. It tends to occur more frequently in women who have not borne children. The pattern of occurrence in some families also indicates that there may be hereditary factors involved as well. When treated early by surgery, or a combination of surgery and radiotherapy, there is a high cure rate.

The majority of these carcinomas arise from either duct epithelium or acinar (alveolar) epithelium (Fig. 11-15). The cells are small, cuboidal in shape, and actively proliferating (Fig. 11-16). They may be arranged in strands or masses and occasionally tend to form glandular or tubular structures. A characteristic of most breast tumors of this type is the dense fibrous connective tissue stroma (framework, or matrix) surrounding the malignant epithelium. Very often, the microscopic picture will show more connective tissue than tumor. The fibrous tissue is not a part of the malignant growth, but a reaction of the body to the rapidly multiplying and infiltrating neoplastic cells. This appearance of fibroblastic (and also lymphoid) elements in the proximity of a growing tumor is called the *stromal reaction.*

Cancer of the breast usually spreads by invasion of regional lymph nodes (the axillary nodes are most commonly affected), and from there to the pleura and the lungs by way of lymphatics. Metastasis through blood vessels to distant organs also occurs.

12

Male reproductive system

The male reproductive system consists of a pair of male sex glands, the testes, which produce spermatozoa; a group of ducts for conveying the sperm cells outside the body (epididymus, ductus deferens, ejaculatory ducts, and urethra); accessory glands that form seminal fluid, such as the prostate and the seminal vesicles; and the external organ of copulation, the penis.

TESTES

The *testes* are paired oval organs, each suspended by a spermatic cord in the scrotal sac outside the body cavity. This cord is a fibrous muscular structure containing the ductus deferens and the blood vessels, lymphatics, and nerves that supply the testes. The *scrotum* is composed externally of integument and is lined internally by a serous membrane derived from the peritoneum. The testes descend from the abdominal cavity into the scrotum during the eighth month of fetal life.

Seminiferous tubules

A thick two-layered capsule of connective tissue surrounds each testis. The outer layer, or *tunica albuginea,* is dense fibrous elastic tissue; the inner layer is composed of vascular loose areolar connective tissue. Fibrous septa (partitions) extending into the gland divide it into wedge-shaped lobules. Each lobule contains one to four seminiferous tubles, which are highly convoluted (coiled) and about 80 cm in length.

The *seminiferous tubules* are lined by specialized stratified epithelium, known as *germinal epithelium,* that rests on a basement membrane (Fig. 12-1). Male sex cells originate from this epithelium. These cells can be seen in varying stages of development, from the most primitive cells *(spermatogonia)* just above the basement membrane, to the mature *spermatozoa* at the uppermost layer lining the lumen of the tubule. The layers in between contain sex cells in intermediate stages of maturity. The spermatogonia on the basement membrane are round, light-staining cells. They divide by mitosis and produce cells of the next layer, the large *primary spermatocytes.* The primary spermatocytes divide by meiosis (reduction division) to produce smaller *secondary spermatocytes* which quickly divide and differentiate into even smaller

106

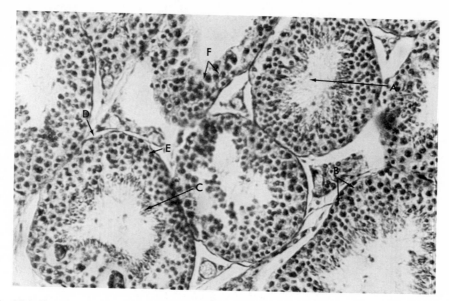

Fig. 12-1. Testis, cross section of seminiferous tubules. *A,* Lumen of tubule, *B,* Sertoli cells, *C,* spermatozoa, *D,* basement membrane and lamina propria, *E,* spermatogonia, *F,* interstitial cells of Leydig. (X100.)

spermatids. The spermatids transform by the process of *spermiogenesis* into motile spermatozoa, each of which has a *flagellum* (tail) and a head containing a dark-staining condensed nucleus.

Also present on the basement membrane are scattered tall columnar cells, called *Sertoli cells,* which extend through the epithelial layers and reach the lumen of the tubules. These cells have an irregular nucleus with a large well-defined nucleolus. Large numbers of spermatids attach themselves to the Sertoli cells, which are believed to be nutrient and supporting cells.

Interstitial cells of Leydig

Individual seminiferous tubules are separated from each other by a loose connective stroma that contains clusters of the interstitial *cells of Leydig.* These are round or spindle-shaped cells with large nucleoli. Many of these cells contain in their cytoplasm large rod-shaped protein crystalloids, the *crystals of Reinke.* The interstitial cells are the endocrine portion of the testes. They secrete the male steroid hormone *testosterone,* which controls the development of the secondary sex characteristics and the normal functioning of the accessory ducts and glands of the male reproductive system. *Gonadotrophic hormone* (interstitial cell–stimulating hormone, ICSH) from the adenohypophysis (anterior pituitary) is necessary, in turn, for the normal functioning of the interstitial cells.

The testis is therefore both an exocrine and an endocrine organ. As an exocrine gland it secretes spermatozoa (male sex cells) into ducts. As an endocrine gland it secretes testosterone into the blood stream.

DUCTS

Spermatozoa pass from the lumina of the seminiferous tubules to the outside by way of a complex series of interleading ducts.

The first of these ducts are the *tubuli recti* (straight tubules) and the *rete testis* (testis network). These are thin-walled ducts lined by simple cuboidal epithelium.

From the rete testis, the spermatozoa pass into small ducts known as the *ductuli efferentes*. These are lined by pseudostratified ciliated columnar and cuboidal epithelium, and contain a connective tissue lamina and a layer of smooth-muscle cells.

The ductuli efferentes join with the *epididymis* (ductus epididymitis), a highly coiled tube about 5 meters long. The epididymis lies outside the testis on its posterior surface. It is lined with pseudostratified columnar cells that have long microvilli extending into the lumen. The epithelium rests on a basement membrane, beneath which is a thin vascular lamina propria and a layer of smooth-muscle fibers.

The epididymis straightens out finally and merges into the *ductus deferens,* which is about 40 cm long. It is lined by epithelium similar to that of the epididymis, but the microvilli tend to disappear. The lamina propria contains many elastic fibers. A thick muscularis, composed of three layers of smooth muscle, surrounds the duct. The outermost coat, or tunica adventitia, is composed of fibrous connective tissue.

The ductus deferens rises into the pelvic cavity through the inguinal canal. It crosses the ureter, and at the posterior side of the urinary bladder it dilates to form the *ampulla,* which has a wider lumen and a thinner muscularis than the rest of the duct. Just below the ampulla, the duct of the *seminal vesicle* joins with the ductus deferens to form the *ejaculatory duct,* a small tube about 0.3 mm in diameter and 19 mm long. This short duct runs through the prostate gland and opens into the prostatic portion of the urethra. It is lined by pseudostratified or simple columnar epithelium that has a secretory function. The wall consists mainly of fibrous connective tissue.

ACCESSORY GLANDS
Seminal vesicles

Seminal vesicles appear as elongated sacs with a deeply folded mucosa. The epithelium of the mucosa is composed of pseudostratified columnar cells that contain yellow pigment granules and colorless vacuoles. These cells secrete some of the components of seminal fluid. Below the epithelium is a vascular lamina containing elastic fibers, a smooth muscle coat, and an adventitia composed mainly of elastic connective tissue.

Prostate gland

The prostate gland is composed of branched tubuloalveolar glands embedded in a stroma of mixed fibrous connective tissue and smooth muscle fibers (Fig. 12-2). The

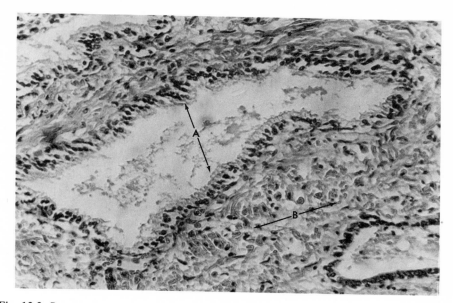

Fig. 12-2. Prostate gland. *A*, Alveolus lined with simple columnar epithelium, *B*, fibromuscular stroma. (X100.)

glandular epithelium is simple cuboidal to columnar and contains secretion granules. The prostate surrounds the urethra as it leaves the urinary bladder, and empties its secretion, a thin milky alkaline fluid, into the prostatic urethra.

Bulbourethral glands

The bulbourethral glands, also called *Cowper's glands,* have ducts that enter the cavernous portion of the urethra. They are compound tubuloalveolar glands lying just below the prostate. Each gland is divided into lobules by connective tissue septa. The secretory acini are composed of simple cuboidal to columnar epithelium. The excretory ducts are lined by simple to stratified columnar epithelium. The outer walls of the ducts contain fibrous tissue and a thin layer of smooth muscle. The glands secrete a clear viscous fluid.

PENIS

The penis has both urinary and reproductive functions. Externally, it is covered by skin. Internally, it is made up of three cylinders of cavernous tissue running the length of the organ. These consist of the paired *corpora cavernosa* (cavernous bodies) and the single *corpus spongiosum* (spongy body, also known as the corpus cavernosum urethrae), in the center of which lies the urethra, the outlet for both semen (the fluid containing spermatozoa) and urine. The corpus spongiosum terminates at the end of the penis in a cone-shaped enlargement called the *glans penis.* Overlying the glans penis is a circular fold of skin called the *prepuce.* Each corpus is enclosed in a fibroelastic sheath, the tunica albuginea, in which strands of smooth muscle can be seen.

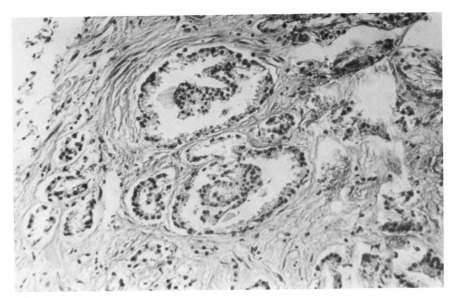

Fig. 12-3. Well-differentiated adenocarcinoma of the prostate. Acini are of moderate to large size, arranged in a random manner, and invading the fibromuscular stroma. (X100.)

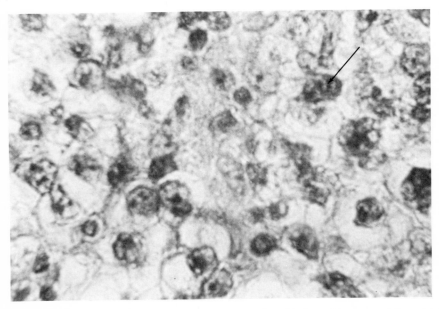

Fig. 12-4. Seminoma of the testis. Sheet of clear cells with large bizarre nuclei containing prominent nucleoli. Mitotic figure (*arrow*). (X400.)

The cavernous bodies contain the erectile tissue of the penis. Erectile tissue increases in size and becomes rigid by becoming engorged with blood. The internal framework of the cavernous bodies is formed by trabeculae (supporting beams), which are extensions of the tunica albuginea. The trabeculae form the partitions and support for large numbers of sinuses, or spaces, into which special helicine arteries open. The sinuses are lined by endothelium. The blood flow into the sinuses is controlled by nerves of the autonomic nervous system, which can either dilate or constrict the arterial vessels. In response to sexual excitement, the vessels are dilated and the sinuses fill with blood.

The structure of the male urethra is described in Chapter 7.

TUMORS OF THE MALE REPRODUCTIVE SYSTEM
Carcinoma of the prostate gland

Tumors of the prostate gland occur most frequently in men in the seventh and eighth decades of life. They may coexist with a benign hypertrophy (enlargement) of the prostate gland, which is common in men past the age of 50, although the two conditions are probably not causally related. The male urethra is surrounded by prostate tissue, and benign prostatic hypertrophy often obstructs the outflow of urine from the bladder.

The prostate gland consists of glandular epithelium and a stroma composed of fibrous connective tissue and smooth muscle. Hypertrophy of the gland occurs when both the glandular and the stromal elements increase. Adenocarcinoma arises only from the glandular epithelium (Fig. 12-3). The malignant cells are generally cuboidal or low columnar in shape, and the tumors tend to be well differentiated; that is, they may form distinct acinar and tubular structures closely resembling the normal architecture of the gland. The malignant acini are somewhat irregular, however, and invade the fibromuscular stroma in scattered groups.

The tumor characteristically metastasizes through the blood vessels to the bones of the pelvis and the spine. Spread to regional and distant lymph nodes is also common. Regression of the primary tumor, as well as the metastatic tumors, can often be brought about by estrogen therapy.

Seminoma of the testis

Seminoma is a relatively uncommon tumor occurring in younger men and frequently affecting *ectopic testes* (testes that have failed to descend into the scrotum from the abdominal cavity during fetal life, a condition known as *cryptorchism*). The malignant cells are derived from the epithelium of the seminiferous tubules and may resemble spermatocytes or spermatogonia. The tumor consists of sheets of closely packed large round cells, with clear cytoplasm and large nuclei containing a single nucleolus (Fig. 12-4). There is usually very little stroma. As the tumor grows, it replaces the normal tissue of the testis.

Metastases to lymph nodes and to distant organs such as the liver and the lungs usually occurs by way of blood vessels.

13

Endocrine glands

Endocrine glands are ductless glands that secrete substances called hormones directly into the blood stream. Hormones are chemical activators, controlling many vital functions of the body. The endocrine system includes the hypophysis (pituitary gland), pineal gland, thyroid, parathyroid, suprarenal (adrenal) gland, gonads (ovary and testis), and pancreas (islets of Langerhans). The gonads are part of the male and female reproductive systems and are discussed in Chapters 11 and 12. The pancreas is a dual exocrine digestive gland and endocrine gland and is described in Chapter 5. The other endocrine organs will be considered here.

HYPOPHYSIS (PITUITARY GLAND)

The *hypophysis* is a small round gland, resembling a grape, that lies in the *sella turcica* of the *sphenoid bone* at the base of the skull. It is connected to the *hypothalamus* (a part of the diencephalon of the brain) by a stalk, the *infundibulum,* and is enclosed in a fibrous connective tissue capsule that is part of the *dura mater* of the brain. The structure of the gland is complex and consists of two major divisions visible to the naked eye, the adenohypophysis and the neurohypophysis. The *adenohypophysis,* in the anterior of the gland, is composed mainly of specialized glandular epithelium. The *neurohypophysis,* in the posterior of the gland, is a firm white tract made up of nervous tissue that has extended downward from the brain.

The adenohypophysis is further subdivided into a *pars tuberalis* (a cuff of epithelial tissue around the stalk), a *pars intermedia* (intermediate lobe), and a *pars distalis* (anterior lobe). The neurohypophysis is subidvided into the *pars nervosa* (posterior lobe) and the infundibular structures. In man, the pars intermedia, which lies between the pars distalis and the pars nervosa, is undeveloped and the pars tuberalis appears to have no specific endocrine functions.

The human pituitary hormones are derived from the pars distalis, or anterior lobe, and the pars nervosa, or posterior lobe. These two lobes, which make up the bulk of the hypophysis, are functionally two distinct endocrine glands.

Pars distalis (anterior lobe)

The pars distalis is the largest portion of the hypophysis. It is composed of a parenchyma (functioning tissue) of cords and clusters of epithelial cells in a delicate stroma (supporting framework) of reticular connective tissue. The parenchymal cells of the pars distalis are either *chromophils* or *chromophobes,* based on their affinity for stains (Fig. 13-1). The chromophilic cells are subdivided into *acidophils* or *basophils,* depending on whether their cytoplasmic granules are stained in reddish or bluish tones with specific dyes. Acidophilic cells are round or oval, with generally abundant pink to orange granules. There are at least two acidophilic subtypes that secrete growth hormone (*somatotrophin,* STH) and *prolactin* (lactogenic hormone). Basophils are larger than acidophils and have fewer granules, which generally stain blue. There are several basophilic subtypes that appear to secrete *thyroid-stimulating hormone* (TSH, thyrotrophin), *gonadotrophins* (follicle-stimulating hormone [FSH] and luteinizing hormone [LH], which in the male is also known as interstitial cell–stimulating hormone [ICSH]), *adrenocorticotrophic hormone* (ACTH), and *melanocyte-stimulating hormone* (MSH). The chromophobes are pale-staining cells with few or no granules. They are believed to be inactive chromophils that have discharged their secretions.

The pars distalis is highly vascular. Interspersed between the cords of epithelium is an extensive network of sinusoidal capillaries with wide irregular openings lined by reticuloendothelial cells. The sinusoids are the second capillary bed of the hypophyseal

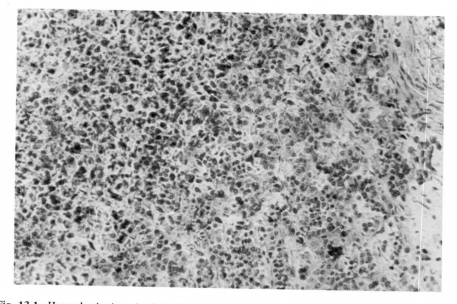

Fig. 13-1. Hypophysis. Anterior lobe showing chromophils (dark-staining cells) and chromophobes (light-staining cells). (X100.)

portal system. The first set of capillaries in the portal system is in the pars tuberalis and the infundibulum. The two capillary networks are connected by portal veins running through the infundibulum. The first capillary bed is closely encircled by nerve fibers from the hypothalamus. These nerve endings from the brain secrete various releasing factors into the blood flowing to the pars distalis. In this manner, the brain appears to control the secretory activity of the anterior lobe cells.

The intermediate zone (pars intermedia) in man is continuous with the pars distalis. In this region, basophils and colloid-filled sacs lined with low columnar cells can be seen.

Functions of the adenohypophysis

Seven hormones are produced by the adenohypophysis. These are trophic hormones, which have widespread effects on other endocrine glands and on target tissues throughout the body. For this reason the pituitary gland is often called the master gland. Growth hormone (STH) stimulates body growth, particularly the growth of bones. Prolactin stimulates the secretion of milk from mammary glands after parturition. Thyroid-stimulating hormone (TSH) regulates the secretions of the thyroid gland. The gonadotrophins (FSH and LH, or ICSH) initiate ovulation and the formation of the corpus luteum in the female, and regulate the output of testosterone by the interstitial cells of the male testis. Adrenocorticotrophic hormone (ACTH) controls the growth and activity of cells of the adrenal cortex. In man, an excess of melanocyte-stimulating hormone (MSH) appears to cause dark pigmentation of the skin. The physiologic significance of this is not known. In amphibia (such as frogs), MSH is secreted by a well-defined pars intermedia and regulates pigment distribution in the skin of these animals.

Neurohypophysis

The neurohypophysis is made up mainly of unmyelinated nerve fibers arranged in irregular bundles that are surrounded by septa of loose fibrous connective tissue and networks of capillaries (Fig. 13-2). The fibers are the axons of neurons of the *supraoptic* and *paraventricular nuclei* of the hypothalamus. (In the central nervous system, a nucleus refers to a group, or cluster, of nerve cell bodies.) About 50,000 of these fibers form the *hypothalamohypophyseal nerve tract,* which courses through the infundibular stalk and terminates in the pars nervosa. Scattered among the nerve endings in the pars nervosa are small specialized neuroglial cells called pituicytes. The nerve fibers of the neurohypophysis contain accumulations of colloidal granules known as *Herring bodies.* The colloid appears to be composed of the two posterior lobe hormones, *oxytocin* and *antidiuretic hormone* (ADH, or vasopressin) in combination with protein. The hormones are actually manufactured by neuron cell bodies in the supraoptic and paraventricular nuclei and are transported down the axons to be stored in the posterior lobe. The hormones are released into the blood by neural stimuli.

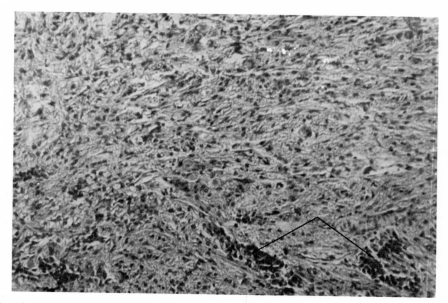

Fig. 13-2. Neurohypophysis. Nerve fibers laden with dark masses of secretion, the Herring bodies (*arrows*). Small nuclei of glial cells (pituicytes) are scattered throughout. (X100.)

Functions of the neurohypophysis. The antidiuretic hormone (ADH) controls the amount of water in the urine excreted by the kidney. It is released in response to a rise in the osmotic pressure of the blood, and causes increased reabsorption of water from the urine in the distal tubules and collecting ducts. In the absence of ADH, large volumes of dilute urine are excreted, a condition known as *diabetes insipidus.* Oxytocin is known to stimulate contraction of the smooth muscle of the uterine wall during during childbirth and also appears to be responsible for the ejection of milk from the lactating breast by causing contraction of the myoepithelial basket cells in the mammary alveoli.

PINEAL BODY

The *pineal body* is located in the roof of the third ventricle of the brain. It is subdivided into lobules by septa of connective tissue that extend inward from the capsule formed around the gland by the *pia mater.* The parenchyma is composed of large clear *neuroepithelioid* cells with long processes that terminate in bulblike endings. The parenchymal cells have been shown to contain large quantities of the biologic amines *serotonin* and *melatonin.* In addition to these cells, there are dark-staining neuroglial elements called interstitial or supportive cells. In man, flakes of mineral deposits (pineal, or brain, sand), composed of calcium carbonate mainly, begin to appear in the gland at puberty and increase thereafter. There is some evidence that secretions of the pineal gland may regulate the activity of the gonads in man.

THYROID GLAND

The thyroid gland is located in the neck and consists of two main lobes lying on each side of the trachea, connected to each other by a narrow isthmus. The gland is made up of many small sacs, or *follicles,* which contain a clear jellylike material called *colloid* (Fig. 13-3). The follicles are lined by single-layer epithelium and are surrounded by a richly vascular loose connective tissue stroma. The height of the epithelium and the amount of the colloid in the follicles vary with the activity of the gland, which is controlled mainly by thyrotrophin from the anterior lobe of the pituitary. When the gland is inactive, the cells are squamous to low cuboidal, and the colloid is abundant. During hyperactivity of the gland, the cells are tall columnar, and there is little colloid.

The colloid in the thyroid follicles is composed of the main thyroid hormone, *thyroxin,* in combination with protein. The resulting compound, *thyroglobulin,* is a temporary storage for the hormone manufactured by the follicular epithelium.

Within the basement membrane beneath the follicular cells there are a few sparsely distributed large clear cells called C cells. These cells secrete the hormone *calcitonin.*

Functions of the thyroid gland

The thyroid hormone, thyroxin, increases the oxygen consumption of many tissues of the body and thus has a profound effect on the metabolic rate. It is also necessary for normal growth, maturation, and mental activity.

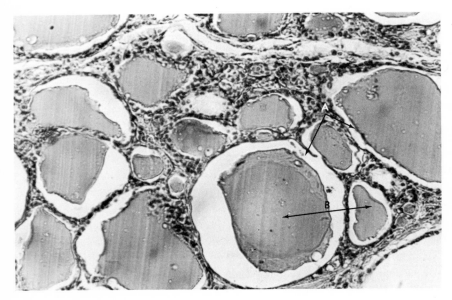

Fig. 13-3. Thyroid gland. *A,* Follicles, *B,* colloid in follicles. (X100.)

Calcitonin lowers the level of circulating calcium in the blood. Its action counterbalances that of the parathyroid hormone.

PARATHYROID GLANDS

There are usually four small oval parathyroid glands embedded in the surface of the thyroid gland. Each gland has a thin connective tissue capsule that dips into the interior of the gland, forming septa between irregular lobules. The epithelium of the gland is very dense and is arranged in plates or cords embedded in a fibrous stroma containing many blood vessels and fat cells. Two types of parenchymal cells are found, the more numerous *chief cells* and the *oxyphil cells.* The chief cells are clear and light staining, with a large centrally located nucleus. The oxyphil cells are large acidophilic cells with relatively small nuclei. Cells that appear to be transitional forms between these two types are also found.

Function of the parathyroid glands

The parathyroid glands produce the hormone *parathormone,* which is responsible for maintaining the plasma calcium at a constant level of about 10 mg per 100 ml of blood. The hormone is secreted in response to lowered levels of calcium ions in the blood and acts by mobilizing calcium from the bones. The parathyroid glands are necessary to life; their removal or atrophy results in *hypocalcemic tetany* and death. A functioning tumor of the parathyroid glands can result in excessive demineralization of bone and *hypercalcemia.*

ADRENAL (SUPRARENAL) GLAND

The adrenal gland consists of a right and left gland resting on the upper surface of each kidney. The adrenal gland, like the hypophysis, is functionally two distinct glands. The outer epithelial adrenal cortex, which makes up the bulk of the gland, has a yellow appearance due to the presence of fatty substances in the cells. The reddish-brown inner portion, or adrenal medulla, is part of the sympathetic nervous system.

The adrenal gland is enclosed in a fibroelastic connective tissue capsule, from which strands (trabeculae) penetrate down to the medulla and merge with a stroma of reticular fibers. A rich network of capillaries and sinusoids surrounds the cortical and medullary cells.

Adrenal cortex

The cells of the cortex are arranged in three layers: an outer zona glomerulosa, a middle zona fasciculata, and an inner zona reticularis (Fig. 13-4).

The *zona glomerulosa* is the thinnest of the layers and lies directly beneath the capsule. It is composed of columnar cells arranged in oval clusters. The nuclei are small, and the cytoplasm contains a few lipid droplets.

The *zona fasciculata* is the widest of the layers. The cells are large and cuboidal in

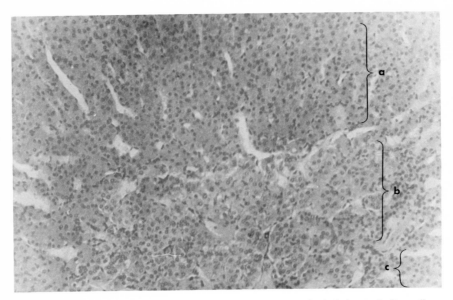

Fig. 13-4. Adrenal gland. *A*, Zona fasciculata (cortex), *B*, zona reticularis (cortex), *C*, small area of adrenal medulla. (×100.)

shape and tend to be arranged in long parallel strands, or *fascicles* (small bundles), which radiate from the reticularis to the glomerulosa layers. These cells have numerous coarse lipid droplets composed of fat and cholesterol in their cytoplasm. Lipid is present in all the cells of the cortex but is most abundant in the cells of the zona fasciculata. The fatty material is often dissolved out during histologic processing, giving these cells a spongy *vacuolated* appearance.

The layer closest to the medulla is the *zona reticularis*. The cells are smaller than those of the fasciculata and are arranged in an irregular network (reticulum). The cytoplasm contains a few fine lipid droplets and many yellow-brown pigment granules that are believed to be accumulations of fatty waste products.

Adrenal medulla

This portion of the adrenal gland occupies a small area in the center of the gland. It is composed of bundles of polyhedral or spherical cells surrounded by a profuse capillary network. The medullary cells are called *chromaffin cells* (having an affinity for chromium salts) or *pheochromocytes* (dark-staining cells) because they contain cytoplasmic granules that turn brown in bichromate solutions. This is known as the chromaffin reaction, and is due to the presence of the catecholamine hormones, epinephrine and norepinephrine, in the granules. Unmyelinated nerve fibers of the sympathetic nervous system end on these medullary cells. Stimulation of the nerves causes the release of the hormones into the blood stream. The chromaffin cells thus function as specialized ganglion cells of the *sympathetic nervous system*.

Functions of the adrenal gland

The adrenal cortex is essential to life. It produces many steroid hormones that can be grouped, in terms of biologic activity, as glucocorticoids, mineralocorticoids, and sex hormones. The *glucocorticoids* are represented by the hormones *corticosterone* and *cortisol,* which are synthesized by cells of the zona fasciculata and zona reticularis. These hormones regulate carbohydrate, protein, and fat metabolism in the body and also play an important role in the body's reaction to stress. The principal *mineralocorticoid* is *aldosterone,* which is secreted by cells of the zona glomerulosa. This hormone is responsible for the maintenance of the water and electrolyte balance of the body. Small quantities of *estrogenic* (female) and *androgenic* (male) *steroid sex hormones* are also secreted, mainly by cells of the zona reticularis.

The activity of the adrenal cortex is controlled by the pituitary hormone ACTH. However, aldosterone secretion is influenced by changes in the volume and electrolyte content of the blood.

The adrenal medulla produces the hormones *epinephrine* (adrenalin) and *norepinephrine* (noradrenalin). These are *catecholamines,* which are secreted at many nerve endings in the nervous system, particularly nerve endings of the sympathetic nervous system. These amines are therefore classified as neurotransmitter substances, or neurohormones. The sympathetic nervous system is mainly concerned with emergency responses, and epinephrine may be considered an emergency hormone. Among other things, it increases the blood glucose level, accelerates the heart rate, and raises the blood pressure.

ENDOCRINE TUMORS

Because of the widespread physiologic effects of hormones, any enlargement (hyperplasia) of an endocrine gland or functioning benign tumor of the glandular epithelium (adenoma), which causes excess secretion of one or more hormones, can result in severe disturbances of body functions. Endocrine disorders of this type are too numerous and complex to be described in detail, but mention can be made here of some that are well known. These include *acromegaly, gigantism,* and *Cushing's syndrome,* which are caused by STH and ACTH-secreting adenomas of the adenohypophysis; *thyrotoxicosis,* or Graves' disease, which is caused by diffuse hyperplasia of the thyroid gland; and the *adrenogenital syndrome,* which is caused by adenomas of the adrenal cortex.

Adenocarcinoma of the thyroid

Thyroid carcinomas often arise from solitary adenomas of the thyroid gland (Fig. 13-5). The tumor cells are derived from the follicular epithelium and may be well differentiated, forming follicles that closely resemble normal thyroid tissue. The less differentiated follicular adenocarcinomas may show little or no tendency to form follicles. These tumors contain islands of solid epithelium seperated by fibrous connective tissue strands. Spindle-shaped cells and bizarre giant cells are often present.

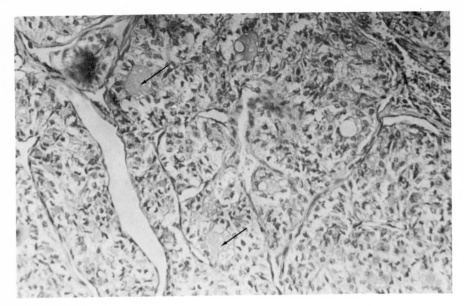

Fig. 13-5. Carcinoma of the thyroid gland. Malignant cells in closely packed follicles separated by thin fibrous strands. Atypical follicles containing colloid (*arrows*). (X100.)

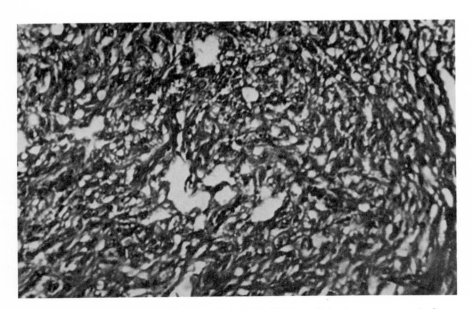

Fig. 13-6. Pheochromocytoma of the adrenal medulla. Highly cellular tumor composed of masses of dark bichromate-stained cells. (X100.)

The tumors spread by local invasion to surrounding structures, and metastasize to bones, the lung, and the liver.

The thyroid hormone contains iodine, and the thyroid normally concentrates large amounts of iodine in its colloid. Well-differentiated thyroid tumors often take up significant quantities of radioactive iodine. In such instances, radioactive iodine may be used for the diagnosis and treatment of the tumors.

Pheochromocytoma (chromaffin cell tumor of the adrenal medulla)

Pheochromocytomas are uncommon tumors that may be benign or malignant. They arise from the chromaffin cells of the adrenal medulla. Pheochromocytomas are highly vascular tumors consisting of islands of large cells with abundant cytoplasm and irregularly shaped nuclei (Fig. 13-6). The cell masses are separated by numerous capillaries and fine strands of connective tissue. The tumors secrete epinephrine and norephinephrine and show a marked brown chromaffin reaction with bichromates. The excess secretion of cathecholamines causes dramatic clinical symptoms, characterized by periodic attacks of severe hypertension, palpitations (tachycardia), headache, excessive sweating, pallor, and anxiety. Surgical removal of the affected gland is the treatment of choice, although patients with pheochromocytomas are often poor surgical risks. Cerebral hemorrhage and coronary occlusion are frequent complications of pheochromocytoma.

Index

Tumor(s), 22-27
  of adrenal medulla, 120, 121
  benign, 22
    functioning, of endocrine glands, 119
    of ovary, 94
    of uterus, 95-96
  of bone, 39-42
  of bone marrow, 42-44
  of breast, 105
  of cervix, 97
    Papanicolaou test for, 97-101
  emboli, 23-26
  of endocrine glands, 119-121
  of gastrointestinal tract, 65-67
  growth of, 22-23
  of kidney, 86
  of liver, 72-73
  of lung, 80
  of lymphoid origin, 56-59
  malignant, 22-23
  metastasis of, 23-26
  nomenclature of, 26-27
  of ovary, 94-95
  of pancreas, 73-74
  of prostate gland, 111
  scirrhous, 23
  of skin, 31-33
  stroma of, 23
  stromal reaction in, 23, 105
  of testis, 111
  of thyroid gland, 119-121
  of urinary bladder, 86
  of uterus, 95-96
Tunica
  of hollow organs, 18
  of vessels, 18
Tunica albuginea
  of ovary, 87
  of testis, 106

U

Unicellular gland, 19-20
Unipolar neuron, 16
Ureter, 84
Urethra
  female, 84
  male, 84, 86, 109
    cavernous, 86
    membranous, 86
    prostatic, 84, 86

Urinary bladder, 84
  carcinoma of, 86
Urinary system, 81-86
  kidney, structure of, 81-84
  tumors of, 85-86
  ureter, structure of, 84
  urethra, structure of, 84, 86
Urine, formation of, 81-83
Uterus, 90-93
  carcinoma of, 96
  cervix of, 92
    carcinoma of, 97-101
  endometrium of, 90
    phases of, 91-92
  glands of, 90
  leiomyoma of, 95
  myometrium of, 91
  perimetrium of, 91

V

Vagina, 93-94
Valves
  ileocecal, 64
  of lymphatic vessels, 50
  of veins, 46
Vasa vasorum, 45
Vasopressin, 114
Veins, 45-46
Vessels
  blood; see Blood vessels
  lymphatic, 50, 52
  structural plan of, 18
Vestibule, of external genitalia, 94
Villi, of small intestine, 64
Volkmann's canals, 35
Vulva, 94

W

Water, exretion by kidney, 83, 115
Wharton's jelly, 7
White blood cells; see Leukocytes
White pulp of spleen, 55-56
Wright's stain, 48

X

X-rays, effect on lymphoid tissue, 56, 58

Z

Zona fasciculata, 117-118
Zona glomerulosa, 117-118
Zona reticularis, 117-118